WILL FERRELL SAVED MY LIFE (...AND GOD HELPED)

ONE MAN'S GUIDE TO SUICIDE PREVENTION

B.L. IYVER

ISBN 978-1-0980-8047-1 (paperback)
ISBN 978-1-0980-8048-8 (digital)

Christian Faith Publishing, Inc.
832 Park Avenue
Meadville, PA 16335
www.christianfaithpublishing.com

Printed in the United States of America

INTRODUCTION

I have worked on this book gradually over time; but most recently, with the outbreak of coronavirus in the United States, I've learned that suicide rates may soon be on the rise. The economy is struggling, unemployment claims in the US topped forty million last week, and, unfortunately, the global death toll continues to rise. This is enough of a reason for me to wrap up my writing and share what I have. As my sister remarked last month when I gained enough courage to share that I was working on a book about my battle with depression, "If your book saves even one life, it will be worth it."—So it is time.

After years of struggle contemplating life versus death, I have come to the definitive conclusion that living with depression is better than dying from it. I choose to live. In your definitive moments of choosing, you must remember that what happens is your choice and no one else's. Please choose life. You are here for a reason, whether you are able to recognize it right now or not.

CHAPTER 1

To My Eldest Son

What kind of man cannot stand and go to the
bedroom door when on the other side awaits a
four-year-old boy who builds his life and dreams around you, his hero.
What kind of hero cries because I cannot play and
laugh when the shadow comes over me.
I know I am your hero. Don't see me like this, clutching
the blanket and crying because I can't hold you.
Ten feet away behind the door calling, "Dad, Dad,"
and I cannot come to you. I am so sorry,
you will never know how sorry I am to abandon you in this moment.

June 9, 2019. As I watched my high school senior wait for his row to be called to make his way to the stage to receive his high school diploma, the thought actually entered my mind: *I made it. I'm sitting here, and this is real. I never gave up, and I made it. I am not dead.* Now, how morbid is that to even think about at your child's graduation? Quite morbid—or quite not, depending on your life situation. In fact, how very real and common a thought that is to those of us who fight this fight every single day.

I am a man who suffers from severe depression and anxiety, so much so that on more than one occasion I have viewed suicide as the better option to my continued suffering and the suffering I have caused to those I love. I am writing to tell you, or better yet to persuade you, that suicide is *not* the better option. Those are common words and easy for anyone to say, I realize, but I ask that you give me a chance to explain because I too speak from a level of experience that understands and respects the type of pain you endure.

By the way, I want to clarify that the use of the term "you" throughout the entirety of this book will always refer to *you*, the reader. While I do not know you personally, I do hope to reach you.

A Charmed Life—Why So Depressed?

When I sit back and reflect on my life, I find I have everything I've dreamed of having in life and am incredibly blessed for it. How is it then that a person like me can have everything I have hoped for and still have the audacity to be "unhappy"? I have struggled with this question for nearly three decades now. Fortunately, I am still here to tell you about it—unlike so many unfortunate individuals who've pondered this same difficult question but are no longer here among us. Because I am here, I have something to say about it. My testimony may or may not help you, nor those in your life who do their best to survive living in the midst of your struggle, but I want to try. What harm can it do to share? If nothing else, it will be therapeutic for me. That's a selfish thought, I know. But honestly, my true hope is that the relevance of my path to survival will help you with your own. That's not too selfish a motive.

Realists

There are optimists and pessimist in this world, and somewhere in between there are those of us known as realists. While we can lean toward the side of pessimism and cynicism, we realists truly do believe in and crave all that is good—so long as it is real. I have only been able to survive my depression and anxiety because I stay real about both. I am not cured. I am not beyond or above my depression, and I am not without anxiety. I do not pretend that either are gone. I can't tell you all the answers, but the story I share may lead you to some answers for yourself. I certainly hope you will give my account a fair chance. I hope to benefit you the way I have benefitted from the stories of others.

The Beginning—Growing Up

I remember being a regular kid in a regular family. No money to speak of, but we had all we needed and did what we could— and we did a lot. So much talent in one household, seems we had a pretty good gene pool. My parents produced a family of small-town star athletes, prom queens, honor-roll students, and general over-achievers. Seven children from two parents who stuck it out together 'till death had them part. Like so many did in those days, my parents stayed together despite regular conflict and daily dysfunction that surpassed that of Archie and Edith, Fred and Wilma, and even Homer and Marge. That's right, a typical blue-collar family. In our home, love and nurturing took a backseat to tough love and survival of the fittest. I remember receiving attention here and there but also an overall consistent lack of affirmation. Compassion was something we did not know, because we did not experience it. There were no hugs, no daily "I love yous," and definitely no tolerance for tears. Uprooting was common, and I remember living in eight different houses before graduating from high school. Nevertheless, I was strong enough, smart enough, and talented enough to make my own way; and that's exactly what I did.

While growing up into my teen years, I was a fairly happy adolescent. I was insecure like most teens, but I had friends and was very involved in school, sports, and other activities in high school. I remember starting to hear a bit about people with significant emotional problems, and I started to recognize that not all people were as emotionally capable as others. In fact, I learned that some people struggled mightily in life, but I can't say I understood at all. I also don't remember truly sympathizing much either. I was too busy with my own teenage struggles in trying to find normalcy. I was already becoming a survivor. I think I actually recognized the struggle of others my own age as something I could use to surpass them and, more so, strengthen my own standing among my same-aged peers.

Like I said, I was the youngest of seven from a family of competitive siblings in a financially modest household. I made it through high school in one piece and looked forward to seeing the world I had not yet seen!

By the time I was in college, I heard of this condition called depression, an actual disease people seemed to have. It was more than being "crazy," it had something to do with whether a person could function or not emotionally. It did not make much sense to me at the time. Why would anyone have that as part of who they were? College was the best of times, so why would anyone be struggling? As a young college student who was discovering life outside of my own small town, it seemed my ego grew proportionately to my new knowledge of the larger world around me. Both grew a lot in fact, and in retrospect, that was not such a good thing. As my ego grew, so too did my acknowledgment and concern for others shrink considerably. I pegged people with the condition of depression as being "messed up," weak, and certainly lower than me. In my twenty-some selfish and competitive mind, I did not have to worry about them. So much for empathy. Their pitiful plight gave me resolve in knowing, "Not me."

By the age of twenty-two, I viewed depression as not only a weakness, but an excuse. I perceived it as a type of ingratitude in others. *Complainers*, I would think. *They think they have it rough? Please. What a cop-out.* And to add to my cynicism, some of the kids I met in college who suffered from a clinical diagnoses of depression came from families that had money—serious money! *Spoiled brats*, I thought. They owned beautiful cars and traveled to places that I had barely heard of. How then could they be depressed? The audacity.

Well, if you are reading this book, then you already know that depression does not discriminate by privilege or economic status and money certainly doesn't prevent it. In fact, I've seen money make it worse. Money can buy lots of temporary fixes, but money is not stronger or bigger than depression or anxiety. And the audacity I insinuated as being inside of others who were experiencing real problems was unfair and unfounded. The only person displaying audacity was me. But I could not see that at the time. By the age of twenty-five, my judgmental side and ego were stronger. As far as life went, I was in it for myself and no others. While this might not be uncommon for people of that age, I am not proud of who I was at that time. We are all shaped by who we were and who we have become, so I cannot spend time in regret but only learn from my mistakes. What's that saying?—"Judge not lest ye be judged." That's exactly right.

My late twenties were quite a whirlwind, and I'd say I was having the time of my life. Living in Chicago during the Michael Jordan era was quite something. Chicago is a great city for twenty-some-things, and I had a blast! But as I ended that decade, there were clear signs of problems with my emotional state of mind. I'll go into greater detail where helpful in later chapters, but for now I just want to help you trace your own steps of how you got where you are today. It's not easy looking back, but it will be helpful.

Diagnosed

By my early thirties, when I was first diagnosed by a medical professional, I remember that day when I saw my own terrible weakness looking back at me squarely in the mirror. I was devastated and confused. My sadness at having to recognize there was something wrong with me that for the first time in my life I could not fix on my own was too much for me to bear. Sadness mixed with confusion, it was my first taste of real desperation. The awareness of my new shortcoming eventually turned from confusion to anger. I wasn't sure whose fault this was. Who to blame? How long had it been brewing inside me?—If I remember correctly, I think I was most angry at myself when I was first diagnosed. How dare I be depressed when I have such an awesome life! What unbelievable right do I have to be down, complaining, melancholy, unmotivated when my life is great! After all, I considered my life easy by comparison to others. I stewed about my diagnosis endlessly. I felt selfish, guilty, and, above all things, ungrateful. What right do I have to be depressed about anything?"—Ungrateful and feeling guilty for it: nice combination. Feeding depression with guilt: a perfect recipe for affirming and sustaining one's misery. There's definitely something important for you to learn from this, and I want to help you unearth this notion.

What Is the Purpose of This Book?

During the twenty-five years since my formal diagnosis, I have learned several things that can, and do, make my depression and anxiety significantly better; and in doing so, I have identified those things that absolutely make it worse. I will try to share as many of them as I can with you. Hopefully, in doing so, I will be giving you a sort of road map to avoid as many of those land mines as possible as you walk down the path you have before you. We men always struggle to ask for directions, you know, but please don't in this case. Good thing GPS came along. Now men only have to enter a destination. No need to ask for directions—God forbid. This book can be a GPS for you, and the destination will be your continued life.

Depression Is Part of Me

Feeling weak, shameful, and ungrateful, depression has its way of setting in like a big, fat, firmly-nested tick. It reminds me of the green phlegm goblin with the suitcase in the Mucinex commercials that moves in to strike down that poor soul with the bad head cold, but then leaves begrudgingly by the end of the commercial when the medicine moves in. At least they have a cure for that condition. Hmmm…medicine. We'll come back to that topic later. For now, remember what I said—depression sets in like a firmly-nested tick. And when I use the term "depression," I'm not talking about being moody or upset here and there. I'm talking about something with much more permanence. Meaning, if your depression is real, then it's not going anywhere. You are going to need to deal with it, and you can.

Part of You

Let's get right to it. If you are reading this book, you are likely already at a point of hoping to save yourself or at least you know you need to change something sooner than later. Maybe you need to change your outlook, your approach, or, most certainly, your outcome. Those of us with depression know we can be taken to the brink at any time. When ending your life feels like the best possible outcome, you need to change that. If depression or anxiety, or both, are part of you, it doesn't have to be the end of your world—or your life. You have options. One of which you already know is, in fact, taking your own life. From my own suffering and overcoming, I beg you to reconsider other options. You do not know me, and I do not know you. But I may know your heart if you struggle as I do. You are not alone in your struggle. Therefore, you do not need to be alone as you fight it.

My List—My Plan

As struggling men, we often feel a need to keep our struggles to ourselves. I am done with that. I want to help others. Considering the depth of my struggle, I can see now that my life has actually gone relatively well overall in these past twenty-five years. Over the duration of two and a half decades since my diagnosis, through trial and error, failures and victories, and some fortunate happenstance, I have developed a collection of practices and strategies that have kept me alive and functioning.

I speak of things I changed in my life over time in order to change my life outcome. Life or death? I always wanted to live, even when I felt I no longer could. As I look at my list of survival strategies, I recognize that each one came from my struggle and fight to sustain over all these years. They are coping strategies—if you will, practices—I learned over time that I have used to outsmart and hold off the tendencies of my own depression. I say "outsmart" because today as I write this I cannot truly say that I have overcome or beat my depression. As much as I wish I could say I have left it behind, that would be a lie.

A Realist's Plan

The plan I've developed is not a panacea nor a snake oil. Like I said earlier, I am not cured. Living with my depression has not been a harmonious coexistence. I am still not completely in synch with my inner self. I have not gotten to know myself through meditation, yoga, or other practices that work for many. Those require a level of patience I do not possess. No, my practices for survival came from bare necessity. Change and survive, or stay the same and die. Those were my choices. That is where my plan came from.

Why Right Now?

Some would probably share their plan at the end of the book as a culmination of ideas, but I share it now for two specific reasons. One, it's an example and proof that there is something concrete to be gained from taking the time to read this book. And two, I share it now in order to demonstrate and admit early on that this plan isn't intended to be the prescribed answer for anyone else but me. It's not the cure for you. No, this isn't meant to be a ten-page book. You can't just read the plan and be done. For people who have already tried one hundred different things to survive living with depression, I owe you the blunt truth. To write "here is the solution" as I present my plan would be to tell you this book is no more than garbage—and it would belong there too. Rather, I share my plan early in this writing so that if there are any type A pragmatists among you, you might find some hope in it and stay engaged. Perhaps, like me, you lack patience and need a hook to keep you connected.

The Plan Is the Key

Many people make plans to commit suicide, but I believe very few people make a plan to survive *from* suicide. Why plan for one and not the other? Think about that. If you have spent time planning all the parts to your death, you are likely a measured person. Therefore, you owe it to yourself to plan for a different option—call it plan B if that helps. Smart people always have a plan B. And I am sorry there is no simple fix to this disease, no single remedy—no silver bullet. You need a combination of supports that work for you. At least give yourself a chance by planning for your survival.

Your list, your plan for survival, will be your own; and it will need to develop over time. Feel free to take any items from my plan and use them. Save time, and in doing so, you might just save yourself. After you make your plan for survival, implement each practice one at a time and you will see positive changes. You may even want to chart your changes in some written format so that you can prove to yourself that something good is happening. When you get to the point where you recognize and understand your plan as being complete, then it will be up to you to decide how you can successfully implement it in all its parts together and, most importantly, how you will stick with it. That will be your list. Your proven strategies. Your plan. Your best chance. You can do this.

Here is my plan.

My list of strategies to live and survive with depression and anxiety:

1) *(No. 1 is not missing by mistake!)*
2) Take the medication—depression is a disease, not a habit or weakness you can break or overcome through sheer willpower.
3) Whether you are more afflicted by depression or anxiety, or both, set aside your pride, lay down your ego, and ask for help or you won't make it.
4) Stop drinking alcohol—period. And while you're at it, stop any recreational drugs you are using too. They are all depressants. Alcohol and depression don't work.
5) Go to work daily. Keep your job, your income, and your insurance.

6) When you are not working, remember the things you enjoyed doing as a child and start doing them again, no matter what they are. Your mind and heart will remember.

7) If your work does not involve service to others, find a way to serve others outside of work.

8) Accept and pay for counseling to understand two things: (a) it's not your fault and (b) depression is a condition you have to acknowledge in order to manage, not a weakness to be ashamed of.

9) Don't wear your depression like a banner, but don't hide it from those people who are important to you either. Concealing it will crush you—and them. Flaunting it will drive others away.

10) Find healthy physical outlets. Pent-up feelings can be dangerous to yourself and others.

11) Don't ever be fooled by the deceptive comfort of isolation.

12) If you are in a long-term relationship, let the other person know what you deal with. And never, ever hold the other person responsible for making your depression go away.

13) Don't ever give up, no matter how much sense it makes to you or how dreadfully exhausted you get. Know and accept that your depression and anxiety will come and go—possibly forever. Plan for it.

Well, that's my list. I love reading it because, for me, it has become my undeniable plan for survival. And it does work. It truly works despite all the challenges and unpredictable aspects of my depression and anxiety. Is it a miracle? Maybe.

So What!

So—big deal, right? Anyone can write a list. And anyone might guess what would be on such a list for people with depression or anxiety. And just because it's written down doesn't mean it will work. Yes, that's true. But my plan is not a common sense guesstimate of what should work. I did not sit down by myself or with a counselor one day and develop that list. I am a survivor. That list took twenty-five years to come together. Through my very personal struggles, I chose one thing here and another thing there until I knew the plan was complete. Only now can I look back and see what has made the cut and what didn't and what it took to realize and accept each piece. I am grateful for the insight and wisdom I have gained. All of my suffering, though, I would happily give back. Suffering for nearly three decades to create a plan. Why?—I want to help others build their plan sooner. While it is true that what did not kill me during all those years probably made me stronger, I would add that the amount of misery experienced by me, and those closest to me, could have been decreased had I acted sooner. I am encouraging you. Make a list, develop your plan, make it comprehensive, and follow it. Whether it takes ten months or ten years, think of it as a winding river that will eventually lead you to the same desirable destination—life over death! A better life for you and, as importantly, for those around you.

You Need a Plan

Set down your ego. Set aside your pride. Do not fear weakness. Do not be like I was. Accept yourself and accept that you need a plan.

Pride

Pride is a road to nowhere, a bridge suspended
in nothingness for eternity.
Pride is all that is ugly, limiting, self-defeating, self-serving.
Pride is indignant, blind, absent of righteousness.
But pride and inner strength are not the same thing.
One serves the self while one serves all others.

CHAPTER 2

You've gathered by now that this book is written in the format of a journal, not so much a manual. While I do explore each area of my plan, there is no specific order. In recent years, I have written about topics as they came to me and you will find a cross section of similar accounts that do not follow any particular order or pattern per se. I write about things when they are most real to me, because it is at those times when they hold the truest meaning for me. Because of that, this account may get confusing now and then. I apologize. Perhaps you'll need to read it twice. I wrote this book in the order I did because it is what makes sense to me. In realizing this, it is also my hope that someone could read it and understand something that most others in my life cannot. Depression is both complex and complicated. It has no certain path or order, therefore leaving others hopeless to relate. That is why I believe many of us suffering from depression often feel so alone. So this book too must have no certain order.

Not Alone at All

My goal from this point forward is to provide you with an open and clear lens into my struggling mind, as one example of so many struggling minds in our world. Enter if you dare. It's not easy reading. Whether you suffer from the same afflictions or not, my sharing in great detail can help you to better understand. Sharing helps me to feel more understood as a person too, which would be helpful. Furthermore, and most importantly, I would be very pleased if my writings made others with this affliction feel more understood in their own right. Feeling understood is a saving grace.

Affliction?

That's right, I said "affliction." And I mean it. Affliction is defined as "a cause of persistent pain or distress; misery." There is something aggressive and persistent about depression and anxiety. For some of us, it is not just a condition we carry with us and manage like an occasional recurring rash. No, many of us are deeply afflicted. I have fought this affliction for years. What I have learned is that, for me, surviving is not about the fight alone. No, surviving is about understanding my afflictions more than it is about fighting them back all the time. I will try to dissect that for you. There is great value in channeling some of the energy elsewhere that you now use for fighting. This affliction is draining. Do you dream of respite from the daily fight? Would you give anything for a good night's sleep? What would it feel like not to be so tired all the time?

A Struggling Mind

The stream of consciousness in the mind of a person with anxiety and depression is burdensome, confusing, and most of the time exhausting. I have tried to research and recognize the traits shared by people with depression and anxiety so as to make this affliction more understandable on a larger scale. But I cannot. On the contrary, what I have learned is that depression and anxiety are not the same in any two people. Yes, we share common struggles and common labels, but our innermost struggles are not shared. No two of us are afflicted quite the same. However, I would submit that it is possible the same strategies can be used to manage these unfortunate conditions. There is a ton of research out there lending an element of truth to this idea. That research has helped me to trust accepting treatment.

Marginalized?

People with depression or anxiety may be diagnosed and treated as one group. Yet both are still unique to each person, so labeling all of us the same has marginalized the reality and depth of our pain. It is hard to all be slapped with one common label that ignores our very personal individual struggles. And I believe common labeling can actually compound the harm of depression specifically. When you are depressed, no one quite understands your personal situation, nor will they ever be able to. That realization, in and of itself, can be the most devastating realization in a depressed person's difficult life. In fact, it is possibly the thing that makes some choose to end it. After all, it is a paralyzing feeling to constantly experience aloneness if you are not seeking it. If no one understands you, you feel alone. If people tell you they understand you but they actually don't, you can feel even *more* alone. And labeling you the same as the depressed person next to you, that is marginalizing. But I have learned to accept the labeling of my condition because over time it has helped me more than it has hurt or marginalized me. My depression and anxiety will always be intensely personal to me. Nothing will change that. But I've gone from being selfish and guarded about it to being glad to pull it from within, name it, and address it. I don't want it after all, so why should I protect and guard it? Just let it go. That's right, let it go. (Those words are *so* much more than just an annoying song—which I happen to *still* like by the way.)

Having survived for years, I've learned something about my afflictions. Although truly debilitating, they don't have to be forever. I am living proof—literally. I state this right now because I know this material is starting to get heavy. Like the weight of living with depression, reading about it isn't easy either. If you need a break, please take one, but come back when you are ready. It's okay to take needed breaks.

Depression

Invincible, superhuman, tall, fast, strong, unrelenting,
bound and determined, righteous,
principled, loving, loved...
You take all of that away.
I hate you with every fiber of who I am.
Where do you come from, why do you come at all,
what possible good do you do in this world?
When you take everything away from me and
make me weak, afraid, small, frozen,
secluded, withdrawing inside myself.
Could never go deep enough and could never hurt more.
Through a lens I see you, but what you see is not me right now

CHAPTER 3

Blame

I don't need you.
I don't need you, and I don't need you either.
I am strong. All I need are the few people who really
love me. You are not one of them, neither are you.
Maybe you all brought me down this time. Maybe it's your fault.
Isolate, be independent, don't let them spread me thin again.

Being Ready

I have taken many breaks between writings. Sometimes an hour, sometimes a day, a week, or even a month. I write when I feel compelled to do so. Otherwise, I don't. To reiterate, that's part of the reason you will find random, or even repeated topics and themes addressed in my writing. While the chapters or sections may be only pages apart, in life they may have been years apart in the making. Thank you for forgiving the randomness.

Misery Loves Company

We are going to move into more personal reflections—for you, they may be profound, trivial, meaningful, or meaningless. It depends on your situation. Let me first emphasize—your situation is *your* situation. I don't understand your situation, only parts of it because we do likely share some things in common. But I hope my reflections help you and others in some fashion by touching upon the commonalities among us. Commonalities can be affirming. If another person affirms the notion that you are not crazy for how you feel, you might feel more sane—and less alone. That's a good thing. Misery loves company? No. In this case, misery *needs* company. As much as those of us suffering from depression or anxiety want to be alone, that is not advisable. It's important to remember that. Whether the melancholy or the resentment that accompany depression and anxiety bring you to a place of feeling you should be alone, try not to buy into it. It's not safe for you. Find company.

The Resentment

How does one explain or understand the type of resentment that comes through having severe depression or anxiety? After all, the thought process is not always rationale or sensible. Let me try.

A resentful person, which I can be at times, might say something like this after reading the first twenty pages: "This book is nothing." Sure. Maybe. Because you can still say in this very moment, "No one understands how I feel, what it's like, who I am, how I got this way, or what my problem is. A book isn't going to change that." And you may further say, "Do not judge me and do not compare yourself to me." And while you're at it, you might even tell me to mind my own business or, conversely, to "Get a grip. Sit up. Suck it up." After all, we all have problems. Problems—ahh yes—none of us is more privileged than others in that category. You're reading this book, so you were probably dealt the cards in life that many would not want. Most likely, you have resentment about it too. Can a book change that? The answer is, I do not know. But I hope it can. You see, resentment is the corrosive emotion that reinforces all of the worst tendencies of a depressed or anxiety-ridden persona. At one point or another, I feel I have resented almost everything and everyone in my life. I've even blamed others at times for things that, in reality, are only inside of me. That's because depression can have an ugly, nasty, warped complexion when your emotions turn bitter over your situation. Resentment for having depression, resentment for whoever or however I got it, resentment for the medicine I have to take every damn day as a reminder that I am not whole without it, and resentment over being so incredibly tired all the damn time. That's right. Don't patronize me or think for one moment, just because I am well enough to write a book, I don't know how bad it gets: How all you want is to be alone. How everyone gets on your nerves. How you're tired even after sleeping all night and all day. And when you can't sleep, your mind runs like a high-speed train that's lost its brakes, just like a gerbil's wheel that spins with anxiousness and worry that simply…will…not…stop. But the biggest form of resentment is that resentment I feel when, no matter how good I live or how many healthy choices I make in my life, my depression and anxiety still will not leave me. So, yes, I do know. Our affliction is not exactly the same, but some of the challenges and emotions that come with it are. And those emotions are destructive, painful, and sometimes much stronger than me. You bet I resent that. I resent it every day, and writing this book doesn't change that one bit. Understand?

What I should do is find a way to resent my considering that suicide is *ever* a good or viable option. Perhaps if my better self would resent that enough, the thought of suicide would disgust me to a point where it is no longer allowed to enter my mind.

The Start of Relatability—The Value of a Book?

I too used to think books were useless for helping in any meaningful way. I saw books as static, inorganic, and boring. Boy, was I wrong. The truth is, I read very few books until after the age of thirty, at which time I finally read a few books that started to change my thought process. The first was by Parker Palmer, an educator, in which he not only admitted to having serious depression in his lifetime, but I learned during my reading that he had made it out alive! As a man, I also found other commonalities that presented themselves to me. For example, he talked openly in the book about how others could not truly understand him or his struggles, explained those things that did and did not help him during his lowest times, and expressed true appreciation for how he came out of it still in one piece. Remarkable. Before Will Ferrell saved my life, I think that book saved my life a little bit too. It's called *The Active Life*. Two things happened when I read that book: (1) For the first time since being diagnosed with depression, I felt that someone else understood how I felt and *that* held immeasurable value for me, and (2) I read about someone who suffered very similarly to my own suffering, and yet he had made it out. Not only alive, but as someone successful in life to boot! I felt tremendous hope. That's what that book did for me. It meant something when I first read it, and it still does today. *The Active Life*, it's worth reading if you have time. It could provide an additional dose of relatability for you.

What's Wrong with Me Anyway?

I have asked a thousand times—what in the hell is wrong with me!? I've vacillated between wondering what I did to deserve this to what I must have done to cause it. You can't help but wonder if there must be something. It's a question upon which a person can ponder endlessly. I can't tell you how many hours I have spent questioning that very thing. Most of that time was not constructive or beneficial for me, and I want you to know that. For people with anxiety or depression, that type of thinking—perseveration—is a form of self-punishment and it does not help. And all of that wasted time you will never get back. There's nothing wrong with reflecting, but pondering that leads to perseverating—that's bad. It's unhealthy. It feeds the anxiety and depression. In your plan for adopting strategies to manage your depression, it is a good idea to set specific times aside to reflect when you can. Quiet reflection and meditation can be very healthy, but it's important to be able to recognize when you're reflecting and when, in contrast, you're actually perseverating. For example, when you are confined to your bedroom and lying there in despair, that is not when healthy thinking occurs. Don't ever forget this: when you are low and your depression or anxiety may be deceiving you, that is when irrational thought disguises itself as rationale thought and when perseveration disguises itself as thoughtful reflection. That is when bad decisions are made and dangerous things can happen. If you cannot tell when you have moved into an irrational state of thinking, make a cue card that you can pull out when you are suffering from a bout that has kept you to the confines of your bedroom. The card should say something like, "You are at a low point right now, you do not think rationally when this happens. Just rest. You are not yourself right now. Trust me, you wrote this when you were level and feeling well. Remember, you are me." And then sign it. Sound ridiculous? It's not.

In summary, *do* find time to reflect. *Don't* make time to perseverate.

Level

My baby son—I smell your hair, I feel your soft skin,
I love you now as always a father is blessed to.
How can there be days when depression
pushes my desire to feel you away?
When my depression pushes you away, that is
when my fight and anger take over.
Every time, you (depression) trick me into anger and
hatred. I aim at you and hit everything but you. Your
deceit is victorious yet again.
From here I see your trickery, but when I
am there, sunken low, I do not.
How to know? What to replace it with? How to shorten the stay?
When you are gone I tend to forget you and
very intentionally—who wouldn't?
My trick for you is to let myself remember when I am
well to know how to manage you when I am not.

CHAPTER 4

Going Down

Slipping down, clawing, reaching for light, for anything to hang on to.
Stepping up with my feet like a rock climber, but they just
sink into the mud and I slide down in the sludge.
Soon I am warm, I am covered, I am deceived in comfort.
Leave me alone, let me be. You could not
possibly understand where I am.

Others Want to Help

Try not to get upset with others when they try to help. That's part of the resentment, isn't it? No one knows how you feel. Hopefully, they don't say they do (but often they do say it, I know). You are right, they don't know exactly how you feel. Again, that's because depression and anxiety are different for each of us. We resent others if they say they understand how we feel, and then we resent the same people for not being able to understand. Not very fair to them, is it? Then, ultimately, we move into in a state of guilt for imposing our unfair judgment upon others. It's a killer. Literally. Remember, that's why I'm writing this book. Depression kills. It takes lives every single day. If you think I am overdramatizing this, then you may be lucky enough that you are not so terribly afflicted. Or maybe you are reading this book to better understand someone you are close to who is. Either way, it is not an overdramatization. There is nothing more dramatic than suicide. Don't ever underestimate a person's misery or how painful it can be.

Moving On from Resentment

Let me say it again. The biggest insult anyone can give you is to tell you, in your depressed state, that "I know exactly how you feel." That can hurt. When others who know me best cannot even help me, I feel very alone, even hopeless, because I don't understand how you can know me so well but be blind to my pain. Hopelessness is a terrible feeling. Terrible. I'm so sorry for all of the hopeless moments you, the reader, have had. No, I don't know exactly how you feel, but I have a fairly good idea.

Regardless, you must not give up. I have learned there are special people out there who may not understand exactly how you feel, but they have been trained to help *you* understand how you feel, why you feel that way, and what to do about it. This is usually not your spouse or significant other. And it shouldn't be. That's too much pressure to put on someone you love and who already tries their best to love you back. See a professional, a qualified third party. They can and will help. You'd be surprised at how much it helps just to talk to someone. Even better than that, therapists and counselors give applicable strategies that work. I've found that some of the simplest things they've advised made bigger improvements to my situation than anything I had tried to that point. Remember, when you get help, you have a better chance. It's okay to ask for help, even if you're a strong man at heart.

If you are a person who struggles to seek or accept help, trust me when I tell you that doing so will lighten your burden. Don't believe me? It took me twenty-five years to learn and accept this. Does it really need to take you that long? I want to live. Do you, somewhere inside, want to live? Accepting help will bring another day, and another, and another. I have learned that the morning is always there if I let it be. Whether I sleep or lie awake all night, it comes. "You made it one more night," I have often said to myself in deep relief. Some people will read that statement and not understand what that means in its fullness, but many of you will. If you've never experienced it, consider yourself lucky. When making it through a single night is like climbing Mount Everest with no oxygen, then you will understand. Accept help. Others can and will breathe life into you!

Normalcy

*To appreciate normalcy is to no longer take it for
granted, to know when it is leaving.
To fight the anxiety or at least understand it, and wait
patiently with faith knowing this is not your fault.
Hard to remember in the moment when everything
is wrong and nothing seems without fault.
Where did normalcy go?*

CHAPTER 5

Strong

When I'm strong I see you.
I look in the mirror and I see you there. Behind my eyes.
I laugh at you because now you are weak and I am strong.
I hope it is not just you that makes me strong. All these
years. If you go forever, will I still be strong?
Will I know what strength is? Will I even care?
Will that be, could that be the best day of my life.

Weakness

Remember, it's okay to cry. Tears are healthy. I wish I would have been allowed to cry when I was young. Don't get me wrong, plenty of things happened to make me cry, and I did. It was just not supported. Crying was viewed as weakness or, sometimes, ingratitude. "I'll give you something to cry about!"—we've all heard that one. I wish I could have associated crying with strength and normalcy; it is both of those things. I think two of the healthiest things in life are tears and laughter. I've learned that as I've gotten older. May you experience both in plentiful amounts. (Remember, Will Ferrell can help with the laughter!)

Acknowledging

Acknowledging your real pain is very hard, but it is also very important. I fought and fought to overcome the pain of depression for years, always to full exhaustion. Never to a point of victory, never to overcome the weakness, and never to a point of overcoming this terrible affliction. Trying to rise up, to stay above it. Trying to keep my head above the water. "If I can just do that!"—sometimes it is so hard stay above it. Depression and anxiety can come over you when they choose, and sometimes it's when you least expect it. You don't always see it coming. Sometimes you are ready to fight, but other times you just can't muster the strength. Or sometimes, it's too late by the time you try and you're in the slump already. Too tired to fight. Well, I have learned over these twenty-five years that fighting against depression and fighting along with it are two very different things. If you can fight depression straight on and beat it, then you should. Seriously, I have tried, but I cannot. My own personal experience is that my best efforts set me up for failure time after time. That's because fighting can be a win-lose scenario. In win-lose scenarios, the house always eventually wins due to the odds. I am not the house. I hope to be able to find a way to explain that better in a future chapter because for me, as a competitive person, learning how to fight smarter and not harder has been a challenge against my own nature but also a key to my survival. Repeat after me: "The first big step in being smart is acknowledging my condition, even if I cannot fully understand it. I have to admit I have it." The second step is, stop fighting to a point of exhaustion. That doesn't mean give up, and it doesn't mean you should stop fighting for your survival. As Obi-Wan Kenobi said, "There are other ways." Read on.

Stronger

My weakness is my strength. Depression and anxiety have strengthened me because they have made me resilient. I'm going back to that old adage I mentioned earlier, "What doesn't kill me makes me stronger." With depression, however, I wrestle with the notion that what does not kill me *this* time can in fact kill me next time when it comes again. And that's no joke—nothing petty and nothing slighted. When living is harder than dying, that's when you can really get stuck. But I refuse. I refuse to give up. I love my wife, my children, and my life too much. You have your own loves in your life. Say this with me: "Life is a gift, and I intend to live it. I am strong, damn it!"

Yes, depression and anxiety have strengthened me. But they have also hurt me and weakened me time after time. When they come on, they beat me down like I am nothing. At my lowest points, I am completely incapacitated. I am no longer myself and certainly not who my wife or children know me to be. In my deepest hollow, I am not anything that makes sense to anyone—especially me. Those lowest episodes can be the stuff of deep, dark torment. I thank God that, apart from Him, not too many others have seen me in that state. Only a few. I hate it. I truly, truly hate it. But in my weakness, that hatred uses plenty of emotion and therefore drains me even further. So one day I started thinking, *This hatred of my affliction—there's got to be a way I can use it. Not as a destructive force, but as something else.* Being stuck in hatred and resentment is not the way. It can be a starting fluid to ignite my engine, but it cannot be the fuel. Feeling anger and resentment can seem better than the alternative of feeling nothing, as I sometimes do in my lowest points, but it can't be better because the anger only weakens me further.

Let bitterness get you motivated and moving if you must, but then set it aside. It's ultimately a weakness that will hold you back and get in your way if you keep it out in front of you. Steer with something else once you gain your momentum. Hope has a reliable compass. Set the anger and resentment aside.

Weaknesses or Strengths?

Admitting and accepting our weaknesses leads to recognizing that our weaknesses can sometimes actually be our strengths. It is common for people to hear, "Your greatest strength can also be your greatest weakness." What does that really mean anyway? With depression or anxiety, it might mean that which holds you down may be the very thing that can bring you up. For example, while some people contend that depression is only a symptom of larger problems yet to be uncovered, other experts will say that the depression can be the cause of one's problems. What brings you down and brings you up will be unique to you. To figure it out, you have to be okay accepting your depression as a weakness because it is. That's the only way you're going to start getting help. Remember, help is a good thing. Repeat after me: "I need help, and being able to say so is a strength." I wish I would have been able to say I needed help so many years ago, but I was too ashamed. Please don't be ashamed. Shame hampered me for too long. If you want to live, do not allow yourself to be ashamed of your depression or anxiety. Go ahead and be sad, hurt, resentful, or angry. It's okay. It's even healthy—to an extent. Let your emotions roll. But whatever you do, do not be ashamed by your affliction—ever. Shame is another deceitful part of your affliction that helps it to maintain its hold on you. Don't give your affliction that gift.

Accepting

After acknowledging comes accepting. After years of trying, I fully confess I have not done well to accept my conditions of depression and anxiety. I have resented them since I first experienced them. That was in my late twenties. I can still remember how and when it came to be. I left college, got a job, starting living my own life, and kept partying for about five more years. Then, as expected, I started to grow up and slow down. When I did drink, I started to notice that my hangovers got progressively worse and recovery got increasingly harder. Next, my moods started changing unpredictably. That was very hard for me and my significant other. In fact, looking back I know I refused to acknowledge it for about five more years from the time I first sensed it within me. I thought I could shake it. I worked out like good athletes do, took a few days off from drinking, leveled out. I kept control and stayed above it. The affliction of severe melancholy and burdensome anxiety was a weakness I was not ready to accept. "Not me, not now—not ever." Well, unfortunately, when I

31

decided not to admit or accept that I was struggling, my anxiety and depression notified me. Meaning, if you don't deal with your problems, they will find a way to deal with you. You can't hide from them or cover them up forever.

If you can talk to a professional to determine whether you are suffering from anxiety or depression, you have a better chance of getting good treatment. You know, the right tool for the right job.

It is my belief that my depression grew from untreated anxiety, and yet I did not know or recognize the anxiety within myself. It was certainly there, but I didn't see it. One day it came calling, and it changed my life forever.

Bastard

You are a bastard.
You may have been born in me, you may have been
passed from my father, but no loved produced you.
You are a bastard and will never be more. You are a
pathetic virus. A parasite. Someday I will find what
poisons you and use it.
When you come, I sense you. When you come on strong,
you weigh me down. Then somehow you make me
stay down.
You fool me, you comfort me, you warm me, you protect
me, only you are safe for me—safe in you. I still
know what you are.
Soon I will miss my wife and my children, and I will fight
you back and out of me so that I can be with them
again.
You bastard, you have me now but I will be
ready for you next time you come.

CHAPTER 6

Way Down

*Paralyzed, nothing to be done. Nothing can
be done, nothing should be done.
This is all I am.
Leave me here in my room, under my covers where
I belong. I am my own desperation.
You are like extra blankets on me. Heavier than the ocean
on top of me. The darkest, murkiest part of the
ocean; cold, dark, alone, silent—except for a million
concerning thoughts that flood my mind and paralyze
me right here where I lay.*

Anxiety

As I mentioned, I tried to ignore my depression for about five years after I first sensed it. As a strong person, I'm sure I rationalized it as a phase and I did my best to set it aside and move past it. And like I said, my affliction finally notified me. It was not going to be ignored.

Dizzy...disoriented...tears...why? What is happening? The room is spinning, losing balance, going down to my knees. What is this? Embarrassment, confusion—fear, fear, and more fear. I am no longer in control of myself. How awful this feeling is. Vertigo. Unending tears, no explanation, no understanding. Getting to my bed was the only solution I knew, and hanging on until the room stopped spinning was like the worst seasickness a person could ever experience. This was hell for sure.

I was lucky it happened to me at home. For many, their first anxiety attack happens right out in public. From my understanding, it depends on a person's trigger. For me, I think it was the eventual realization of a failed relationship and the loss of control that came with that. As everything started to change in the relationship, that change eventually meant life as I knew it would be falling apart. My commitment to success and need for control at that time in my life were so great that I could not muster the ability to accept such a devastating failure. But on that day, fixing all that was wrong in my life was not the goal at all. Getting to the protection of my bed was the only objective. Feeling as if I had been drugged, I was not sure if the anxiety gave me the vertigo or if the vertigo came first and led to my collapse. The point is, in my first anxiety attack, I learned that all the things that mattered to me no longer mattered. I was only trying to survive. Everything was reduced to one instinct of self-pres-ervation.—Finally sleeping, thank God. Letting my mind rest. But for three days! Three days with getting up only to get an occasional drink and use the bathroom. Think about the pressure that must have been on my mind, and the release that must have occurred, in order to cause three consecutive days and nights of sleep. I had never been so tired in all my life. It was frightening. I wondered how long it would take until I could get up, how long before I could look in the mirror and figure out what had happened. I knew at that point I definitely had a problem, and I agreed to talk to someone about it. That was probably the best decision I ever made in my life. But how? I was very out of sorts, bumbling, rambling, tearful; and I could not tell you one thing I said when I called. But what that person on the other end of that phone line said to me is what I have, and will, always remember. "You did the right thing by calling. It took a lot of courage for you to call," he said.—Damn right, it took courage! Despite being on the phone in my bedroom where no one else could see me or hear me, I still felt exposed in all my weakness to the entire world. It took a lot of courage for me to make a phone call to ask for help. I remember thinking, *I am completely broken, and I don't know up from down.* Just making the phone call made me dizzy again, and after setting the first appointment to go in and talk to someone, I slept for another entire day.

I remember at that time I was far too confused, private, and ashamed to allow anyone else to make that phone call for me. In retrospect, however, I would tell you to act differently if you have that option. I recommend if you have someone you trust to make the phone call to find help for you, let them do it. No shame. Anxiety can make dealing with a simple phone call, trying to provide insurance information, or even obtaining driving directions completely overwhelming if you are on your own and in a time of intense struggle. That sense of being overwhelmed can stop you from seeking and finding help. You must understand, that phone call can be the difference between whether or not tomorrow comes.

So Now What?

After my first anxiety attack, I found someone to talk to for a few months and I "got better." Going through a professional also helped me to keep my job, even though I needed time off. That was really important because my job provided my insurance. It was also the first time I realized that the trigger for the anxiety attack was only that—a trigger and nothing more. It did not define or encompass the larger issue of me having anxiety and depression. Meaning, although I wanted my problem to be episodic in nature and temporary, it would not prove to be that. But at that time in my life I wasn't ready to accept that reality. Still I remember wondering, *When will it happen again? How will I know? How can I prepare? How can I prevent it?*—And then I did what I always do: I rationalized the situation. After all, rationalizing helps things make sense. Rationalizing brings reason and order. The old me: "I can control this. I just need a break. Some rest. Some exercise. A few drinks, some dancing. Yes. From now on, I will see this coming and will make sure I change direction before it comes over me again." I thought I could prevent anxiety from ever hitting me like that again. For five more years I followed that path, thinking I could control my condition and find ways to make things okay. Much of the time, I could. But not enough of the time. How much time will you take?

After up and down swings for a few years made life more difficult than I could manage, I eventually came closer to acceptance and I agreed to try medication—but reluctantly and only temporarily. That was hard. I didn't want to need medication. While it provided needed relief, it also brought on more resentment and what I learned once I started taking medication only made that resentment grow.

All in the Family

When I informed my sister and mom that I had agreed to try medication for what was defined to me as a clinical diagnosis of depression and anxiety, that is when I found out: there were three other males in my family already dealing with depression, and at significant levels. While it made me feel a little better to know I was not alone, it didn't make me "feel" any better. After all, why hadn't anybody told me? If this was hereditary, then I might be stuck with it forever. I resented that possibility, but it was a place to start. Two of my older brothers were already on medication; but my dad, being from an earlier generation that did not acknowledge the need, was not. He definitely should have been. My poor dad. No meds, no drugs, and no drinking to any degree. How did he cope? I would go on in the years ahead to research and understand several things about depression and whether or not it is hereditary, but I can tell you what I have personally grown to believe. Hereditary or not, it is not required that a person experience depression or anxiety just because one of his parents did. Furthermore, poor patterns of behavior and lousy coping skills in families can create a continuing likelihood for personal emotional struggle from generation to generation, but for my own children's sake, I am hopeful that it does not have to be that way. Perhaps being prone to depression and anxiety doesn't have to guarantee a life with the affliction. However, at the same time, I knew that meant there would need to be changes in my own adult life. Do you recognize needed changes in yours? If you grew up in an emotionally unhealthy family, include that in your counseling. That can help you understand it isn't your fault and move toward forgiveness, which will lift a heavy burden. Hopefully someday, acceptance and forgiveness will overtake any bitterness or resentment you have toward your own family, if you have one. Then you can focus on making the type of changes in *yourself* that will lead to a healthier home life for your own family.

Stress and Family

Just this year, a very wise man told me, "Stress does not come from pressure. Rather, it is a person's response to pressure that does or does not result in stress." Well, that's just dandy. Growing up in my house, pressure *did* equal stress. Period. I never knew any different. If it was that way for you and you never learned to cope with pressure in a healthy way, that's not your fault. But it is your problem now. Changing your mindset on this even a little bit moving forward can help you and your family a great deal. Take time to figure that one out. Pressure does not have to equal stress. Good to know!

Why Do I Have This?

I have asked doctors why I have depression and anxiety and the "choices" seem to boil down to (1) my childhood and upbringing in a household full of daily conflict or (2) a chemical imbalance in my brain. "Well, how did that happen?" is always my next question. While my siblings and I may be predisposed to some sort of chemical imbalance, to which I will concede may be possible, I don't buy it 100 percent. I contend, rather, that my unhealthy childhood homelife is likely the biggest culprit. We learn and adopt what is modeled for us as we grow up. Different people cope with stress and anxiety in different ways. Different people deal with anger, conflict, and deep emotions in different ways too. What I observed daily were the wrong ways. Day after day a collection of unhealthy approaches to coping were stored up inside of me and then finally overflowed. If you share the same reality, find a way to make changes so that it does not have to be passed down—again.

What Is Your Reality?

This is a good time to ask some questions of yourself. Today you may or may be able to answer all three of these questions, but you're going to need to sooner than later:

"Why do I suffer from this affliction?"

"Am I willing to go to counseling as part of my treatment?"

"Am I willing to take medication as part of my treatment?"

Treatment

I never liked that word "treatment." It sounded so medical to me, like there must be something *really* wrong with me if I needed that! But it turned out that I did need it. Had I not had it, I'm not sure I would still be here today. My treatment is part of my survival.

Medication

Medication was quite an experiment for me. Be ready for the ride. If you have not traveled the medication route yet, get prepared. It's trial and error, but it almost has to be. Try this; now try that. Put on weight with this medication; lose all your weight with that medication. You can't sleep with this one, so take this one too in order to rest. This one causes electric shocks if you stop taking it, and be careful because that one might make you suicidal.—Wait, what?— I'm taking something to help me cope with depression, but it might make me suicidal?! What's that all about?

Be Prepared

Within the trial-and-error process of trying to find what medication works for you, it can get challenging and the lack of immediate results can jeopardize your sense of hope, especially if you are trying to work, trying to lead a normal life, trying to stay married, trying to avoid that low dip again—trying and getting exhausted from it. If it takes months or even a few years to get your medication regiment right, it is important for you to know, that is not unusual. Try to be patient and know going in it will not be a quick fix. Give it time. It is worth the wait and worth the continued struggle you'll have to endure while you and the doctor figure out what works for you. In the meantime, try to keep things low key in your life if you can. No alcohol, no recreational drugs.

Be Patient

Now, if you asked me twenty-five years ago to be patient and accept that medication wouldn't be a quick fix, I *definitely* wouldn't have wanted to hear that. I needed help—immediately. But the solutions are not immediate. That's hard. I know how it feels to want to be healthier—to get better. Patience.

Pills

Pills, what sort of thing needs something else in order to be whole?
Almost everything needs something else to
make it whole. But pills? Pills?!
Three times you have kept me. Three times I have
left you. Three times I have returned.
I scorn my need for you like I believe our
public would scorn me if they knew.
Pills can crucify one's character if it lay in judgment
of those who are blessed not to need them.
Pills are bitter reminders of what I can no longer be without them.
Does beating this mean no more pills? I don't think
so, but for now I don't know what ever will.
That realization is a very hard pill to swallow.

CHAPTER 7

Sliding

Sliding, sometimes like a slippery slope. But most of the
time more like a slowly eroding sand dune that
makes way beneath me.
I do not sink into a hole, but rather the perimeter rises up around me.
A fortress? A prison?—An abyss.
There is no deep hole, only walls all around.
Then I am pushed back up, when you decide—or is it when I decide?
I cannot tell which one of us is in control.

Why Am I Here?

We are here on this earth for a reason. Our life is a gift, and so I
ask you again to please not give up. If you feel you cannot withstand your affliction even one more minute, just stop counting the
seconds. Tomorrow will come. It always comes. There were many
nights I could not fathom how I would make it to the next day, but
I did. It just happened. You don't have to give up. You don't have to
give in. You don't have to give your life over to desperation. There
are concrete ways to equip yourself for managing the struggles. I will
continue to share some of those with you right now.

Owning It

After accepting your condition, you must own it. The truth is this: if it is real anxiety or real depression, it is yours. If it is chronic and becomes part of your life experience, don't try to wish it away. And as I've already said, don't rationalize it whatever you do. The temptation to rationalize or label your depression or anxiety so you can neatly file it away might be hard to resist. Good luck. If you can do that, more power to you. But if you cannot file it away permanently, then you are like me. You will need to own and understand your affliction and how to navigate it in order to survive.

Anxiety or Depression?

Sometimes understanding leads to a question of defining. Do I have anxiety or depression? Surely you've noticed by now that I often mention both and, at times, almost interchangeably. For some people I am sure they are not so interrelated. For me they very much are. If they are closely linked for you, knowing which ones follows the other for you may be important. I don't even know which came first for me. What I do know is that if a person can understand what their affliction looks like when it rears its ugly head, then it can be recognized and therefore addressed. As Mr. Rogers said, "Whatever is mentionable is manageable." This means you can be helped. Celebrate that!

Some say anxiety causes depression, and others say depression causes anxiety. Regardless, either can cause a state where a person is unable to cope with anything, making everyday tasks arduous and stressful. If you have never been incapacitated by your emotional state, you're one of the lucky people—because it's just awful. The stress that comes with it is debilitating. Every task can feel stressful; every normal responsibility can feel overwhelming—coated in a shell of intense pressure. It's no fun. What a terrible way to feel every time an expectation arises. I'm sorry if you experience this in your day-to-day life. You do not deserve to feel that way. No one deserves to feel that way. I'm sorry.

Molehills or Mountains?

Anxiety and depression can be compounded over time if untreated, and that is why medication can be a smart path if you need it in order to stay out of or above the incapacitated zone. Both afflictions make molehills into mountains, and those mountains almost always appear too big to climb. So—don't climb them. No one says you have to climb anything. Isn't that a relief to consider?— As I said, there may actually be another way, Obi-Wan. Make your list. Start writing your plan.

Forever a Worry

I knew in the back of my mind after experiencing that first anxiety attack, it would not be my last. In talking to a counselor, I also began to realize that my anxiety had its roots planted quite early in my childhood. Somehow, at some point in my young life, I became a worrier. An overanxious, nervous, insecure, constant worrier. I don't remember when it started, but I think it was when I was just little. Scary movies I shouldn't have seen, my dad losing his temper frequently, a household full of constant yelling, wetting my bed all the time, the insecurities of puberty, trying to measure up to older siblings…who knows what started the problem. But it is a problem—a big problem. Falling asleep to worries. Waking up to worries. That's an awful way to live. Some of you know what I am saying. For those who don't, consider yourself blessed. Just know that and be grateful. There is nothing better than good sleep and waking with a clear mind to start the day. On the contrary, bad sleep and waking in a state of anxiety is a terrible thing. Worry, panic, trepidation, fear, scattered thoughts, envisioning all of the bad outcomes that could happen today, envisioning and feeling each scenario, including the impending failure and trouble of each bad outcome that has not even happened (and most likely won't). "Why do you do that to yourself?" a counselor once asked me. "I don't know," I answered, and that was the truth. "If I knew, I probably wouldn't do it," I added. It's no fun being a worrier. But a man who takes life seriously is bound to naturally have concern for things, isn't he?

Concern vs. Worry

As I have grown older, with help I have learned that having legitimate concern for things is not the same thing as worrying. Furthermore, rationalization and self-justification that concern and worry *are* the same will only lead you further down the rabbit hole. Waking up at 3:00 a.m. with several things on your mind and running over them in your head until getting-up time at 6:00 a.m. often means being exhausted even before the day begins. In plain language, it sucks big time. I have learned there are concrete ways to change that unfortunate ritual of waking and worrying. Here are a few I have learned: change jobs; change bosses; change relationships; stop using alcohol; exercise more than you do; try prescribed medications until you and your doctor find what works for you; and when you sense you are happy and your anxiety is low, write down what you are doing during that week or month, who you are spending most of your time with, what you are eating, what may have made you experience joy...and then take that information to your counseling session and share it. Let a professional dissect it for you. You should not expect to figure all of this out on your own. If you could have, you wouldn't be in this position right now. This is a time I would ask you: are you seeing anything in recent history that has served you well and that could be a start to your list of survival strategies? Jot it down now before you forget. It could be the start of something very important and wonderful for you.

Start Your List

Build a list; make a plan. Keep it simple. Keep what works; get rid of what doesn't. Just one condition: no matter what ideas you get rid of as you develop your plan over time, you can't get rid of *you*. That's not an option. Write down the specific things you do, or experience, that you've noticed put you in a good state of mind, that make you productive, keep you level, and have you getting along with others well. These should be the first things on your list, the start of your plan. Over time you will find that some things were accurate and some not so much. Some things stay on the list; some things drop off. Like the medication, it will be trial and error. Some things you try may even be new practices to replace old ones that did not serve you well. Just because there are things you've been doing forever doesn't make them the right things. It can be really eye-opening when one of those realizations comes along. I found there were a few things consistent in my life for decades that weren't serving me as well as I thought.

My First Attempt at a List

I remember my thought process in starting my first list. I've come a ways since that time, a time when my pragmatic mind thought I could just "program" my cure. Back then I put too much emphasis on controlling everything. Take a look:

Control—isn't that what it's all about after all? I can't control my depression; so I will try to control everything else—my day, other people, triggers, etc. For so long I have tried, and it is exhausting. It is time to look at what I can control, given all other variables and things I cannot control. What can I?
I think I can control these things:

- *Go to work (it's always okay once I'm there)*
- *Choose the time I leave work on most days (it will be there in the morning)*
- *Scheduling exercise twice a week (and doing it!)*
- *Sleeping more in the winter to rest my tired mind and body (even if sleep wants more sleep, at least the angst is less)*
- *Play with my kids (rather than isolate—really important for both of us—they will remember and thank God, so will I)*
- *Keep the house reasonably clean (feels good to look around, one less thing to worry about)*

- *Fruits, vegetables, and lots of fluids (can't hurt)*
- *Do what my wife needs even if I do not feel it is needed (since she cannot "cure" me, which pains her, I know, at least living with me should not be a punishment to her)*

So it was a start. Not a bad first list, but certainly not my final list. In fact, that was ten full years ago. From then to now, I've kept some of it and replaced some of it. There were things I thought were important back then to managing my depression and anxiety that I've learned are not so important. There are other things, conversely, that I did not even consider back then that today are essential in making my life healthier and more stable. You have to start somewhere. That's important. But if I could give you one piece of advice as you get going on this—don't rely on "control" to fix things. Learn from me. It's not about control; it's more about consistency.

Control Is Overrated

Organized and responsible people naturally feel a desire to control a certain amount of what occurs in their daily lives. Control can be helpful in steering life toward positive, desired outcomes—aka getting one's way. I have learned after so many years that control is overrated. While my desire to control lends to increasing the chance of positive outcomes for the situations in which I find myself, that same control can be very tiring as well as lead to outcomes that may not be the best ones available. Control prevents spontaneity and chance, two key ingredients to realizing life. After all, we do not see all outcomes for every given situation simply through our own limited perspective. Control, therefore, is more limiting than liberating. Something to think about.

Up #2

*Waking in the morning, two little ones jumping
on me. Knees in my stomach and chest,
laughter everywhere including from me.
How could life ever be better?
Their smiles, my bear hugs where I never want to let them
go—freeze them in time so they never grow up.
How could I ever feel differently than this?*

CHAPTER 8

Hope

I don't remember what it used to feel like to be free of
concern. How I long to be irresponsible, lazy,
spontaneous—or not; fun, liked, disliked—
but all for being me. The real me.
How can I just be me when I never know when light will
turn dark? When I hold the rails to wait out my
recovery. Thank God people around me love me, you cannot
trick me away from the love I know I have felt.
I know I can feel. I know I will feel again—
because love is greater than sorrow.

The Title

Will Ferrell Saved My Life—and God Helped. I won't be talking about
religion or God until the last chapters, and there is a reason for that.
There are millions of people out there suffering from anxiety and
depression, and I do not want any of you to write off this book
because it has a Christian premise and you simply don't subscribe to
that at this time in your life. You still need help like me, and sharing
in my story may be a way to help. So whether you are Christian or
not, please read on. Remember, it is the relatability factor I am hoping
will help you. Knowing you are not completely alone and knowing
your condition in not completely misunderstood or unrecoverable. It
is very important to know your burden is not insurmountable.

How did Will Ferrell save my life, you ask? Well, Mr. Ferrell, it is the laughter you brought to me, and out of me, that saved me. It is your ability and gift to take me away from my problems during the amount of time you have my attention, and even after that when I think back to your humorous lines and antics, that saves me. I thank you, Will Ferrell, and many other comedic actors whose work has accomplished the same wonderful benefit for me. I thank the writers who provided the material. And as I age, I find more and more truth in the saying, "Laughter is the best medicine." Absolutely. You see, there have been so many times over the past twenty-five years when, sadly, laughter was simply not possible for me. So when it *is* possible, it is gold. Don't ever under appreciate a good laugh. There's science that supports it as being very beneficial to a person's health. They say the chemical release that occurs in the brain when we laugh is very good for us.

So why Will Ferrell specifically? Hopefully not so he will sue me for using his name in the title of my book. Using his name is fitting. It wasn't random at all. Just like every case of depression is unique, so may be its remedy. The fact is, I chose this successful comedic actor for a very specific reason. Several comedic actors who came before Will Ferrell in engaging me and taking me to a better place are, sadly, no longer with us. And it is not due to old age. It is because they gave up on life. Sadly, they were some of the best. I do not know whether or not they had severe depression or anxiety, I just know they died too soon. I would say addiction to drugs or alcohol is a form of eventual suicide, so in my eyes, they all killed themselves regardless of the final action that ended their lives. The bottom line is they just couldn't make it. And I am sure they fought the good fight. Before giving up and giving in, these comedic actors helped me to laugh and at times feel well enough to not give up in own my life. So when they each died, I was both sad and angry. I knew that the lonely, bitter, and seductive darkness had taken them. Whatever it was for each of them—the killing burden, that is—was simply more weight than they could hold up any longer. During the time of my life when these now-deceased personalities did live and shine, their talents captivated me and, in many of their various on-screen roles, engaged me and helped me escape my constant worries. I am so grateful for that. As an introvert, it has always been movies, not other people, that kept me level and often brought me up when I was low. Movies truly take me to a different place. They made me appreciate something better, something outside of myself. And when the talented people I had admired died, I was distraught but empathetic at the same time. I actually felt to a certain extent that I understood. When Robin Williams took his own life, for example, I remember that day. And I remember exactly what I said to my wife only minutes after hearing. "I get it," I told her. "It's so hard. You just get tired of fighting it every single day—day and after day. It's exhausting. I understand why people give up. I do."

But seeing people who appear to be happy and have everything in life suddenly give up, that's confusing for the rest of us—unless you struggle yourself. If you struggle, you know that nothing material, including money nor success, can cover your pain or make you better. Maybe that's what makes life even harder for those with fame, because they feel they should be happy and content but they are not. I mentioned earlier how I experience guilt and confusion around my own depression, because I've experienced a life that should make a person content. But I struggle to feel at peace. It's often hard to tell with others what their emotional state is. Sometimes you can see the signs, but sometimes you can't. In fact, a respected police captain in a neighboring town went to work one morning this year, clocked in, and shot himself in the head, killing himself and leaving his wife and family behind. No one from the community expected it, but perhaps those closest to him may have. It is amazing how some can cover their struggle so well and conceal it from others. But know this— that act of covering will wear you down. Those of us with depression who make great efforts to conceal it understand why people become exhausted. We can understand why people eventually get too tired to try anymore. That's why it's time to stop concealing. It's okay not to cover up. You may have a better chance if you are not weighed down with that burden too. Having depression is hard enough. Spending energy to cover it up all the time can be *too* hard. It can be too much to sustain. Whether it is pride, shame, or fear, find out and unearth it.

The Darkness Beneath

I worry that the same darkness that took the lives of some of my favorite actors and comedians will continue to take more lives—mine included. Maybe if these people only knew all of the happiness and brightness they brought to others, they could collect that light and use it to combat some of their own darkness. And what about Will Ferrell? Well, in my limited knowledge of his off-screen life, there is still something different and very positive about him—or so it seems at least. I never hear about any deep personal struggles in his life or those closest to him. Was it a more stable childhood, a more nurturing household growing up, a stronger marriage, or maybe something else? I would not have any idea. I just know that I do not see or sense the same instability or darkness inherent in those who have taken their own lives when I watch Will Ferrell on and off the screen. Therefore, to me he is truly blessed. Not because he is so talented and successful, but because he appears to have all he had aspired to in life and it hasn't ruined him—or worse yet, it hasn't killed him.

Do What You Love

I believe those who do what they love in life find happiness naturally and that their fame is just a by-product, not a goal. I see peace in them. I yearn for that state of mind. To feel peace, happiness, satisfaction, self-worth, gratitude and contentment. And why not? Isn't that what we all want?

So I thank you, Will Ferrell. You have helped to keep me alive. Part of your purpose is certainly to help others laugh. So there is actually a morsel of truth in me saying you have saved my life because, as I have already expressed, the laughter you create is the best medicine I could have.

My Thing

Those who know me best know that movies have been my escape, my temporary joy, and always a healthy distraction from other things. The escape one can experience in a movie, the awakening of curiosity and wonderment, the amazement and engagement— it's magical. The healthy preoccupation is like that of a good book or a great soundtrack. Do you have a healthy distraction or two? Write down what they are. Make sure you do these things even when, and *especially* when, you are struggling.

Purpose

Will Ferrell's purpose in life is to make others laugh. Can we agree on that? I would like to think that writing this book is part of *my* purpose. I also believe that the essence and contents could not have come at an earlier time in my life. They just couldn't have, because they did not exist and neither did my understanding of all of this. I had to experience the deep pain and confusion that came from surviving and learning through the previous twenty-five years. I do still hope it can be different, sooner, for you. Learn from my struggle. Let that be my gift to you. Let there be purpose in all of this. Let there be one life saved, or maybe more. And let yours be preserved.

Remember Your Plan is Still the Key

I will be sharing my plan in its entirety near the end of this book. Remember, your list of practices and strategies is the key, and that is why it has to be your own. Your plan must be *your* plan, and it should be one that works for you. It would be great if my plan works for any of you, but it is not intended to be that way. And the time your plan takes to develop is yours too, no one else's. But if you can borrow pieces from my list—my plan—please do. I believe some of my strategies may be universal in managing depression and could save you years of unnecessary and wasted suffering. You decide.

The Point?

The point is, I am so close to being exactly where I want to be in my life. For decades I have worked hard, I've survived, I've prospered, I've grown, and, by American standards at least, I have succeeded. It may have been easier to have failed in life, succumbed to addiction or other vices and to then move into depression with a belief that my difficult life had brought it on. But that is not my story. I have a good life, a wonderful wife, and three beautiful children. I'm still here, so you can see I have not given up. You are reading this, and so it is clear you have not given up either. Your courage sustains you. Your love of life and those in it is real. Write down how you feel on your good days so you can read about it when you are down low. It is good to read about where you *will* be even if you are not there in the moment. Sort of like waiting for the sun to come out after the storm. You can picture it. Learn what you can from me. For a man with severe depression and anxiety, I have a solid amount of credible advice based on proven practices and authentic experiences.

Up

Feeling awake
Feeling light
Feeling fun
Feeling kind
Feeling it is OK to be out and about
Feeling—normal
Right now, this is how I feel so this is who I am—today.
Tomorrow?

CHAPTER 9

To My Family

If I knew you would be happy, I would die right now.
So tired, so sad, so unforgiving, so critical, so jealous, so
angry, so greedy, so selfish, so trying—trying to
survive, trying to live, trying to see your face and know I should stay.
So ashamed because I have everything, and yet in my
shadow I have less than the ability to reach outside of
my own dark cavern—small, cold, cozy, alone.
Chained death is security?
Death is Satan's shadow forgoing all the love around me.

Deep Roots

Depression grew within me over time and is now so deeply rooted that nothing I do will kill it, remove it, overcome it, conquer it, beat it, or release it. It is part of me. I hate to say it. I hate to write it. I hate to acknowledge it, admit it, or certainly to accept it. I truly do despise it with every fiber of my being. Even after twenty-five years? Yes.—Why? Because depression, over time, made me hate...myself. And that hatred fed my depression. It fueled the unhealthy emotions that already weighed me down. It is like a virus in me, a gluttonous greed trying to control me and keep me down, incapacitating me at all costs. It's a beast. A big, hairy, ugly, heavy beast. And yet it is part of me. Learning to accept that is a very difficult thing to do. But as I have already stated, you *must* accept it in order to deal with it.

Hating one's self can form a justification for killing one's self. If you are the villain, you can be the hero in the end. Maybe you think others would be better off without you. You think the world would be a better place. You think it will end all the suffering. You think... too much. I say this next statement often: depression is a deceitful liar. Depression can make a bad decision seem like a good one; it can make a single option seem like the only option. Depression can make a person's judgment void of reason, a heart void of forgiveness, and a soul void of feeling. Depression can bring a human being to a point of such intense emotional sterility and barrenness that there is no longer any sense of pain, anguish, or loss. Maybe it is that barren state of mind that makes the act of suicide painless. Maybe it makes suicide incidental. Maybe there is a place beyond despair.

If you happen to ever feel that way, numb to death, make a promise to yourself right now that you'll go to someone and find a way to tell that person. If you have to fight your way out of the bedroom, find a way to do it. If you can't leave the space you're in, use the phone. Call until you reach someone. Text if you cannot speak. Be honest; don't say you are fine. Say, "I need help." You don't even need to know what that means in the moment. If the plea doesn't make sense to you, it doesn't matter. If you are that stoic that you feel death is incidental, then you do need help. When you are your better self, you would certainly understand. And I bet you would gladly help others (and you will someday) who are in that same desolate place. For now, let them help you. Let people serve, because that actually helps them. If you are like me, you were not brought up asking others for help. Because of that, today you may unwittingly be depriving others of the benefit they would get from helping you. But most of all, by not asking for help, you deprive yourself. That is such an unnecessary act.

Colossal

You are like a microscopic bacteria that can kill an elephant.
Depression is colossal, but I know better. I know you
should be nothing, a spec of insignificance.
You are a microscopic fault, one misfired electrical impulse,
not enough sleep, too much alcohol, the wrong
gene.
You are my smallest feature but my greatest weakness.
I am the elephant—colossal and strong. I will stomp
you out. As God is my witness, I will beat you
someday.

CHAPTER 10

Grateful

Grateful that you are letting me be
Grateful that you have been removed—
But I know you are not gone, just resting perhaps
You will never be gone
After years I understand that I can only lessen you,
manage you, respect you, hate you, forgive you...
and minimize your influence over me

Laughter Is the Best Medicine

Yes, Will Ferrell and others have given me laughter. Even when things were more dark than anyone outside of me could ever understand, I could still have moments of laughter. I may not have made a facial expression or any sound, but inside my hurting mind, I was smiling. And because of that, I knew I was still in there somewhere. In those moments, knowing that gave me the hope I needed in order to believe I could eventually crawl out. And it was a crawl. Every time. Something about movies, though, they've always given me something good that I could use. There's a movie for every mood and a story for every time. And when I need to laugh, I turn to Will Ferrell. Be careful when choosing what you turn to. With depression, we can all be drawn to things that seem appealing but are not really good for us. Those can include certain people in our lives or other things we lean on. Here's a nonnegotiable: you can't choose drugs or alcohol.

Alcohol

I reminisce often about my college days. My undergrad experience was a completely different type of education in my life. I was often joyful back then. I laughed constantly, but I also remember that I drank constantly—after all, the drinking age was eighteen. I partied, and I slept—when I wasn't playing sports, that is. There were two things that made me happy in college—sports and partying. Unfortunately, grades weren't in those top two. Yet I think I was happy. I was in great physical shape in college, so that seemed to help keep my head balanced. I was not a good student in undergrad, but I enjoyed my experience greatly. For me, it was one big life celebration and a boatload of student loans I didn't take notice of until it was time to start paying for them!

After college, as I wrote earlier, I partied for about five more years while I worked and discovered the city life—Chicago. While things were pretty good, I had my ups and downs, which became more pronounced over time. I was in counseling and was approached with a new topic I was not familiar with. I had gotten to a point with my anxiety and depression where I accepted taking medication. At that time, I learned the meaning of a new term that struck me with great interest—"self-medicating." As it was explained to me, some people drink alcohol to unknowingly settle the craving in their brain for certain stimulants. Depressed brains crave very specific types of stimulants. Drinking worked for me. Subsequently, that was also about the same time in my life that my body and mind starting telling me, "You can't drink like this forever." But if I was self-medicating through alcohol, now what? My whole social life revolved around drinking. I did stop drinking eventually, but even that process was off and on for several years. The hardest part of ending my drinking days was that I was actually a fun person when I drank. I was happy and free from my worries, and I had a great time. In general, the people around me had a great time too. As an introvert by nature, I was more sociable and likeable when drinking. Saying good-bye to that part of me was hard. And being no fun was, in essence, no fun. But as I experienced more extreme highs and lows, I could not continue drinking. My wife and I decided to bring our first great gift into this world—our first child. I had to level out. Partying no longer worked for me, and that became painfully clear.

Then I had to ask myself, "Had I masked my depression all these years with alcohol? Was I self-medicating?" In other words, did I have depression starting when I was eighteen but not know it because of drinking for those last ten years? Did I have this affliction even before the age of eighteen? Wow—that was a lot to think about. I certainly didn't know the answer and probably never will. What I do know is, when I finally stopped drinking, my highs and lows were reduced to a much more manageable level. If *you* suffer from anxiety or depression, or both, I highly recommend you stop drinking alcohol completely if you can. Self-medicating will eventually break you down, either mentally or physically—or both. Alcohol is a depressant. It is the last step into death for many people suffering from depression. For some it is alcohol; for others it is drugs. Pick your poison, then leave it behind. You'll *never* regret stopping.

Life after Alcohol

My drinking days were over. Eventually, I even learned again how to socialize and actually have fun without drinking. I also experienced something else new and awkward. It can be hard being the only sober one around others who are drinking and getting silly, and it's pretty enlightening too. Egads, was I like that when I drank? These are my friends, whether they are drunk or sober. I did eventually get used to that, and so did they. Most are still friends today.

I can tell you one thing: I don't miss the hangovers. Not one bit. But I miss the good times. Letting go, letting loose. I've had to find other ways to relax, and I am getting there. Baby steps. If you stop drinking, know that you will need to find other outlets you enjoy and that are good for you. Again, think of what you used to enjoy in your youth and turn to those things again. It never fails.

As far as drinking goes, from my own experience, I would offer this: Those who drink to lighten up are probably okay to drink. Those who drink to numb the pain probably shouldn't be drinking at all. For people with an emotional or chemical imbalance, the trade-off between the brief high and the plummeting and persistent low that follows is not an equal trade. The high cannot be sustained over time, and the low is nothing any person would want to sustain. I wonder if this is what creates addicts. The low is so awful that a person will do anything to escape it. But make no mistake, the low will always be waiting. Whether you feed your lows or not is up to you. I have chosen to try to starve my lows. I miss the highs, but I am also working hard to redefine different highs in my life. Doing that requires redefining the meaning of joy. That's been a very challenging thing but a good thing for me. It comes with maturity, and it eventually brings new wisdom.

Adapting to Humility

One day I said to myself, "Hey, I am doing so well without alcohol!" With no longer drinking, I convinced myself that removing alcohol and its affects should afford me the opportunity to stop taking the medication I so deeply resented each time I put it into the palm of my hand and then into my mouth. The daily dose of humility and shame of admitting that I, by myself, am not enough to help myself through this alone. Doctors told me, "Don't feel bad about needing medication." They told me it's no different than people with diabetes who have to take insulin every day. There is no shame or disappointment in that; it is a condition people cannot help. Just like your condition. You shouldn't be hard on yourself about that. But it *is* different, to me anyway. Diabetes is physiological, whereas depression is (I believe) psychological. There is a test that shows when someone has diabetes, and you can see the results clearly in the blood work. There is no test like that for depression or anxiety. So there is no way to feel it is normal or natural to have the affliction. If it was clear that some sort of unavoidable chemical imbalance occurred in my brain that caused me to struggle emotionally, they would be able to measure it somehow just as they measure other medical conditions. But they can't. Not yet anyway. I've seen brain scan images that are starting to gain ground on explaining more about depression and anxiety, but there is a ways to go, I think. You see, I don't just want to get better, I want to understand my condition. However, despite my desire to get better, I have on more than one occasion defeated myself by going off my medication. Please, no matter how good you feel, don't stop taking your meds.

Getting Better

I have seen enough doctors and sat with enough therapists to know that understanding my depression is only part of how a person can get better. It does not work alone. Even they will tell you, the best results in terms of "getting better" are seen with a combination of medication and therapy. Neither of which are free by the way. So if spending money brings you stress and compounds your anxiety, that takes getting over. And when changing insurance plans means changing therapists, you have to get over that too. By the way, "getting over things" is part of the challenge people like me have because of anxiety and depression. While the insurance and medicine are necessities, don't count on the solution to your problems from the ever-changing insurance industry or from your doctors alone. Realize you will have to adapt over time to change, and know that you have to adapt to disruption in order to survive. Disruptions to treatment can cause you to want to give up like thousands of others, so prepare yourself. When disruption in treatment is upon you, tell those you consider to be part of your support group that a time of change is coming for you. That way you are not facing disruption alone and others can help to support and expedite the change on your behalf—whether it be a change in doctor, medication, insurance, or the like. If nothing else, they can at least be more present for you during disruption if they are aware.

The more improvements you make to your life, through the development and implementation of your plan, the healthier you and your discretion will become. You will start to notice that your life and your moods are just a bit more functional and that your days are more productive and level. It's a good feeling. But the better you get, the more tempted you will be to test your discretion. For example,

I was angry that quitting drinking alone wasn't enough to make me mentally and emotionally healthier, because to me it was an enormous sacrifice. I wanted that sacrifice to be enough, to be worth it, to allow me to no longer need medication. It was the right decision to stop drinking, and it is still worth it today, but it did not fix all my woes. I still needed my medications. But I got over it. I'm sure there are people who stop drinking and then no longer need medication to manage their mental and emotional health. That's a good thing. That may work for you, but it did not work that way for me. If you try it, make sure you tell your doctor first. Tell your significant other too, if you have one.

Just One on New Year's Eve

Just one I can deal with and not have depression.
Just one I can work out of my system on a treadmill.
Just one with friends is important to show love.
Just one feels fine the next day—wow!
Added bonuses: Day two agitation and distractibility
Days 3, 4 and 5, scattered-ness.
Plus, if you order now, 5 additional days of self-doubt tacked on.
Just one...hmmm.

CHAPTER 11

Alone

Someday you will go
Someday you will go and never come again
Believe me, you have my blessing to go
You will not be missed
You will never be known, never be uncovered, never
be understood—but I will never miss you
If I could, I would strangle you and take all life from you
myself with the strength I know I have, the strength
I've acquired from fighting you
Will killing you take me?
I have known you for long enough that I wonder
if you will ever please leave me alone.

Like a Shark

You will hear people say the shark is an amazing animal. It is a perfect biological creation, the perfect predator, the perfect killing machine. In my world, depression is the shark—a perfect predator and the perfect killing machine. I am not comparing a shark to depression in a sinister way. Please understand, I have learned to understand and appreciate sharks and their existence. What I am saying, rather, is that depression is just as efficient and self-sustaining as the shark species that has adapted and survived so well throughout history. But sharks are beautiful creatures, so perhaps that's a poor comparison.

Maybe a better comparison to depression would be the cockroach. They're pretty resilient and hard to get rid of. I just saw the other day that scientists are not even sure they can kill roaches anymore. Similar to super viruses that are becoming immune to our medicines, cockroaches are gaining an immunity to even the strongest pesticides. And I've heard they can live on for a week even after being decapitated!? It's truly remarkable and frightening—and gross. So what about depression? Why am I making this comparison? There is a good reason. You can read on, but my intuition tells me this might be a good spot for a break in the reading. You decide.

Breaking Spots

As I indicated before, when I was writing this book I took breaks. Sometimes I would walk away for an hour, sometimes a week, sometimes a month. And I let it be that way. As such, I am suggesting that maybe this book should be read in the same way—pieces at a time. Of course, that depends on you. Do what you want. Do what works for you. All I ask is that if you do walk away, please come back. I say this to you as much as I say it to myself. I hope this world still needs me and is not done with me. I am betting it is the same for you. The further you read into this book, the more involved you will be in the struggle I live. Much like your struggle, the harder the reading may become as you keep going. If any part of my experience is similar to your struggle, while it may not be uplifting to read, I believe it can help. If you need breaks, take them. If you can only read two to three pages in one single day, do that. Don't put pressure on yourself to read this account all at once.

Back to Cockroaches and Sharks

Both will be here forever is what I think—cockroaches and sharks. That is something I am trying to accept about my depression and anxiety. That's the strange comparison I'm trying to make. It is quite possible they may be with me forever—at least in my earthly life. My depression actually seems to adapt in me to survive, and despite doing so much to curtail it, it lives on. I am trying to understand that it doesn't matter whether or not I want it, it is likely going to be here with me no matter what. I have questioned why and would be lying if I said I would ever stop questioning. My goal now is to try to accept the reality of permanence so that I can work with the undeniable cards I have been dealt. I talked earlier in the book about the importance of acknowledging and then accepting. "Accepting" is not actually the term I would use in my case. Honestly, "tolerating" this reality is the best I can do personally. Tolerating and accepting aren't necessarily the same thing, but neither are terrible options. If you can come to peace with your condition by accepting it, then you should. If not, at least tolerate it. Either way, you have to own it. And whatever you do, don't deny it. Your depression and/or anxiety will not be denied. And you will pay dearly if you try to ignore them.

Drop the Straight-On Fight

Are you tired of fighting your depression? I do believe dropping the straight-on fight against depression is a better approach for surviving and coping. What does that mean? Remember, earlier in the book I mentioned the idea of fighting *along* with depression rather than engaging in the endless straight-on fight against it. I will admit, in order to survive, I did need to fight. Depression raises the need to fight, but I'll reiterate that there are other ways. Remember, fights are set up to have a winner and a loser, every single time. Draws are not that common, but I would recommend that a draw be your goal if you are not too proud to allow it. Coexisting with your depression is not a total loss. Not at all. Fight alongside. Try to go with the current of your condition if and whenever you can.

Suicidal Thoughts

I have had suicidal thoughts many times, and I believe these types of events are certainly different and very personalized to every single person, so I do not contend that what I am about to share is meaningful or relevant to you. I would not want to insult you in that manner. Remember, I know how hard it is to have people say they know how you feel. They certainly don't. But those who suffer as you do may have a pretty good idea of what you are experiencing, so don't be too hard on them when they try to relate and help. For those blessed with not experiencing depression, or anxiety, they still do mean well. Always remember, it is hard for people who care about you when they cannot help you despite their best efforts. They need to try, so let them.

I have had suicidal thoughts more during my lifetime while on medication than when I was not on medication. Sound strange? It does to me too. A bit ironic actually. Here is what I can share. I took a few medications that came with a warning that explained, "Using this medication can cause suicidal thoughts, especially in teenagers." I was not a teenager, but that information certainly got my attention. And, well, I experienced it. I will not name the medications here for two reasons: (1) it was my choice to take them and (2) the object of this book is to help people, not to cause lawsuits that will diminish the potential positive impact of these writings. Anyway, I remember being on a medication where I was anxiety-free. At that time, my wife said I was so easy to live with, but looking back, she did say I was a bit sedentary. I remember gaining quite a bit of weight too. I didn't like that part. In any case, my depression and anxiety were being treated successfully and I remember an odd sort of confidence and peace coming over me. Strangely, it was a peace that led me to think about dying and feeling at peace with the notion. So I was not desperate or at my wits' end, I was at peace with the idea of taking my own life. Not just dying, but actually killing myself. It seemed rationale and sensible as a consideration. To think about being at peace back then with taking my own life because of the medication I was on?—That's just plain scary! Those specific medications shouldn't only come with a warning, perhaps they shouldn't be used at all. I am not sure those specific medications are still on the market; that was some years back. If they are, I'm sure they been improved by now. Needless to say, my doctor changed my prescription to something else.

Better Times—Be Smart

While you can see my clear support for medication, I admit during the times in my adult life when I have felt better, when all things seemed to be in alignment, joy was prevalent, and things were seemingly taking care of themselves. Life was good; I decided I was good too. And then I stopped taking the meds. A few times I tried to wean off over a few months, while a couple other times I tried to stop taking one med but still take the other. And one time, I even stopped taking both. Each time, it was not long before I was on the brink again. Rattled, frazzled, uptight, edgy, and anxious. Sometimes it was even worse. If I drank alcohol too, forget it.—Give me the meds! It took at least two weeks to level myself out again after restarting, and luckily, I did not harm myself during any of those periods. Interestingly, in fact, I never felt like harming myself when off meds. But I felt a lot of other negative things, and they were always self-defeating in nature. Thinking back, my judgment during those times of stopping my medications was either plagued with anxiety or steeped in irrational self-righteousness and absolute indignation toward my better self. In other words, I thought I was fine and I wasn't. I thought I was right, but I was wrong. I was above harming myself but not in a healthy way. I was not rationale. I was irrational and sometimes even obtuse. But I could not see it. My wife told me when I was back up and level how hard I had been to deal with during those brief lapses. My poor wife. "Take the meds," they say. And they are right—100 percent right. Take the damn meds.

By the way, I know I keep going back to stories about my repeated decision to stop taking medication over the years and there is a good reason. It is because each time I was so very hopeful, but I was also wrong each and every time. Keep in mind, it is possible that you are feeling and doing so well *because* of the medication. For me, that is the case. No shame in it.

When Medications Don't Work

I have had a few other times that, while on medication, I was still overcome by anxiety, desperation, and hopelessness and I considered ending it. By this time, I had tried many remedies, including medication, and yet I found myself failing—again. That was very scary because I was taking my medication as prescribed, and usually, it worked. I had a wonderful wife and children. During my low points, I often survived by remembering I did not want to be selfish to them, even though I admit I thought they would be better off without me in the long run. I knew I was wrong about that, and something whispered to me just enough to hold me in place. In better times, I am always grateful for the sadness I experience thinking about losing my family because it has always helped me to hang on when I went low. Being able to say, "There is always tomorrow," has become quite powerful to me. Feeling as if tomorrow will never come or when it does, it will be terrible, is so unhealthy for a psyche and so distressing to any human being. I know because I've lived it at least a thousand different times. If it happens too much to you, you're probably not on the right meds, or at least not a strong enough dose of them. And maybe—just maybe—you're not in counseling like you should be. (Notice, I did not say, "Could be.")

If, after a long stretch of feeling good, you start to slip and there is no apparent reason, then it is time to go to your doctor. An increase in your dosage may be needed. Try to stay ahead of it.

If a person is on medication and it stops working, that can definitely be a catalyst for giving up. That almost happened to me. I am hopeful that you have something or someone in your life that needs you more than you can deny. You owe it to them to stay alive. Killing yourself to relieve others of your pain and suffering, and all that comes with it, won't help. You will be passing on the guilt and shame as a parting gift. You could be leaving others asking their entire life, "Could I have done more?" "Why wasn't I enough?" Or worse yet, will they ask, "Is that how I am going to end up?"—Don't do that to them, because I am betting you love them. Underneath all of your anger, desperation, and irrational thought—you still love them as much as they want to love you—if you would, or could, let them. If your current meds are not working enough, take heed.

What's Going On?

There was a time not too many years ago when I was not drinking. I was taking my medications; and I was, by all accounts, level. Then things starting slipping and just kept on going down. I remember taking myself to the doctor and saying, "I am taking my medication, and I still can't function—something's wrong. I don't understand what's happening. I don't want to lose my job, my family, everything. If I hospitalize myself, can they help me?"—I actually wanted to be hospitalized. For the first time in my life with depression, I wanted them to admit me and treat me. I was in bad shape, but still good enough to know I needed help. Good enough to seek help. My doctor said she wanted to try something first. She tested my testosterone level. A normal level was 250–750, she said, with it being common to be over 750 for some men. My reading was 93. Yes, 93! Even I knew that was unbelievable. She asked if she could give me an injection of something right then and there, and I agreed. "I'll do anything to be better," I said. She gave me a shot and asked me to go home and call her the next day. If I had not improved at all by the next morning, she would place me in the hospital for treatment. I was ready to go into the hospital. Maybe they could figure out what was wrong, and at least I could safely rest. But then something incredible happened. After the injection, within hours, my head started to clear up and my mood and energy came up noticeably. I felt less confused, much less desperate, and more level. I wondered at first if it was some odd placebo effect, but it wasn't. I called my doctor the next day, from work where I had miraculously managed to go that morning, and asked her what she gave me. She said it was synthetic testosterone. And upon my requesting, she denied my immediate request for more but said if the injection was helping, it meant that might be the new culprit. Over the next few months we did testing and settled on a monthly dose of injectable testosterone.

Your Testosterone?

For the sake of helping yourself and identifying all the possible culprits to your system, I encourage you to learn about low T. While it bothered me that yet one more thing was wrong with me, I was more relieved and appreciative than annoyed. If you suffer from depression or anxiety, I would suggest you ask your doctor to test your testosterone level. While some conditions affect different people in different ways, I can tell you that low T was dangerous for me. I have had to maintain my existing medications as well, but there is no question the synthetic testosterone has seriously helped me.

Another Failed Attempt

No, I did not try to kill myself and fail. My failed attempt was again regarding my medication. I know it must be hard to believe, but it's true. I share only to help you because some of you will do the same thing!

Once the "miracle drug" of testosterone was helping, I expected to be better. I felt "this is finally it!" I am healed; the culprit was found and addressed. Now I can either start drinking alcohol again and be fun again or maybe I won't be able to drink, but I can at least stop taking some of my other medication! After all, I knew my depression medication made me tired and I also believe they make me heavier. I wanted to shed both of those side effects now that testosterone had made me "better." So like many other men probably do, I tried some things on my own without talking with my doctor. I didn't drink alcohol, but I did stop taking one of my depression medications. Within three weeks, once again, I realized that did not work as I had hoped. All the bad symptoms came over me. So I started the meds back up, and within a week, I leveled out. But hey, if I am going to keep taking these meds, maybe I can at least try drinking again? So after restarting all of my medications, I tried that too. It was awkward at first, but I did laugh and have fun and did not feel too bad the next day. Maybe I had something good here? Maybe I could party again! Maybe I could have just one or two once in a while. But, alas, a few days later after drinking, I sank. It was awful, and I was so saddened. I confirmed yet again that I could not drink and expect to maintain a clear head for the week ahead. I also could not go without my meds without becoming agitated or impatient, so it looked as if I just had to accept needing all of them. I'll say it again, learn from me if you can. Spare yourself the unnecessary lessons.

Dark Horse

Even when I am well, galloping with the strength and
stamina of a thoroughbred, that is when I realize I am
a rope that shortens with every lap.
I see you are the battered hitching post, weathered and
inevitable, and every lap brings me closer to you.
The faster I run, the sooner I am there. Even trying to run
away brings me tightly bound and I am strapped
down to you.
Someday, I will be the center and you will have to run
around me. But then you will stay on the perimeter
in the distant shadows—a dark horse in every sense of the word.

CHAPTER 12

Fire

*Someday I hope to know whether to stomp you out like a
smoldering fire, or light you like a torch drenched
in forgiveness. If I light you so bright that you are
released, can I trust you not to burn me alive?*

Surviving On My Own?

When you are a person who has based your existence and progression in life on the notion of strength, independence, performance, accomplishment, and the like, realizing all the medications that are needed in order to keep you emotionally healthy, is almost enough of a reason by itself to give up. Or conversely, it could be a reason to be grateful. Choose that. If you have a job and insurance, that's huge! I can't even imagine what it's like for those without insurance. Can't treat the anxiety and depression, so hence, that compounds the anxiety and depression. Self-medicating would be the only possibility for survival in my case if I did not have insurance to pay for medication and treatment. That is not to say that all of the addicts out there are self-medicating for reasons of anxiety and depression or lack of insurance, I am just saying it would be a short step for me to go from where I am now to that very place. Desperation and addiction. That is why I judge no one. No one understands the pain and the struggle like those who live it and endure it. And we wish we did not. We wish we could fight it off, forget it, leave it behind.

Again—Why Not Just Fight?

Knowing the depression and anxiety I live with, I cannot succeed by fighting alone. As I wrote earlier, almost every fight has a winner and a loser. That is how fights are designed, and actually, that is their purpose. Competition is for sport. To settle it once and for all. To pick who will be on top and who will crawl away in humble shame. For my entire life, I have fought to succeed and win—as the youngest child; as a person from a modest family who wanted more for myself; as a three-sport athlete who found as much joy in playing as I did in winning; as an overachiever, always accomplishing more or doing more than others expected I might. I have always loved that. I love surprising people, especially after being underestimated. I was built to compete, to fight, to win or die trying. So what of depression—what to do since this thing is real? My natural inclination has always been to fight, of course. And why not, why wouldn't I fight? That has always worked for me. *It will again in this case.* That is what I thought, at least, almost twenty-five years ago when this all began. Surely I can fight this, win, and move on. Someday I would look back and say, "Boy, those were dark days—but that is all behind me now." I used to think I could make it out and leave my depression behind. I'm sure there are those who can. Because I have not been able to, my desire to survive has changed my fight against my depression to a fight I wage on behalf of my plan for survival. I fight for living. If you are a natural fighter, you can still be a fighter but be smart and use your momentum to leverage things in your favor. When you make your list for your plan, recognize the pieces that can work together in supporting you. Direct your fight forward alongside of your depression—not in direct opposition to it. Your plan can help you keep it on a leash.

Using Relatability to Stay Alive

I mentioned earlier that I had read a book by Parker Palmer, and it inspired me because he had made it out of the darkness of depression back into the light. I could relate to the struggles he had written about, and I was so grateful he shared them in such a public and vulnerable manner. I saw hope ahead for myself because, by the time he wrote that book, he was in a much better place in his life. He was the first author I had ever read that talked openly, as a man, about his depression. He did so with no shame, no apology, and no denial. Through reading his account, I could see he had gone into darkness but had somehow come out the other side alive and in one piece. He found a way to survive, and his life went on, successfully. I saw the potential for myself to be next. I could relate to the pain of his experience, and I gained a real sense of hope from learning about his recovery. Some parts of his story were more relatable than others, but there was enough there related to my own experience to help me. I do not know if Parker Palmer went on medication to help him get better, nor do I need to know. His solutions were in his list—his plan. I have my own. But the relatability of his story motivated me to believe a plan for surviving and succeeding was possible. That is my goal for you. It is possible.

The Straight-On Fight—*Continued?*

I know, I know. I said the straight-on fight is not the way. But I am pigheaded, and I must be transparent with you in sharing another one of my faults. Without exception, about every six months I get this thought in my head that I am going to *beat depression once and for all.* I'm just so sick of it, and despite knowing somewhere deep in my mind that I can't actually accomplish it, I convince myself for at least one day twice a year that I can fight it! I get motivated and prepared to fight. Go big or go home! A straight-on fight means all or nothing, and I'm ready this time! With depression as my opponent, I know winning would mean living—"living happy like I used to, feeling like I used to, being who I used to be." Losing, on the other hand, could mean dying. "Losing who I was, forgetting who I am, becoming someone I do not want to be. Why even live anymore?" Losing is dying, figuratively and literally. I wonder if some people with depression end up thinking, *The person I was has died. The person I am is not someone I want to be. It's time for me to die in the physical realm too.*

Suicide. That is an answer, but I'm hoping you see it is not a solution. Life is not a math problem, so we should not consider death through suicide to be a solution for anything. Suicide is an outcome, nothing more, and it is not the right outcome for any of us. Desperation leads us there when we become lost in our sadness—sad for ourselves, our children, our spouse, or our families and our friends. *I will never see them again if I do this, and they will never see me again. Maybe that's best for everyone because I am not the person I used to be*—that's one way to think. My depression leads me to think that way sometimes. But my depression is irrational and deceitful as yours probably is too. I have survived my depression long enough to know that. Know your depression and know it will deceive you. When I start to have those negative thoughts about people being better off without me, I remember and I stop. You have to know better. As far as me being fed up and wanting to beat my depression about every six months—nah, meh, hmmm. I get over it. I do my best.

Losing

Living with depression can feel consistently like losing—or settling. I want to encourage you to look at "losing" as being about growth, not about dying. We learn from our mistakes. When we lose, we get back up and try again. We don't make the same mistake we made last time. We build toward success, even if a hundred more failures come first. It's still growth. What if Edison would have killed himself after nine hundred failed attempts? We'd all be sitting here in the dark! I move forward.

Shame and Guilt with Others

I have learned, for the most part, to manage my behavior in tough times as not to hurt others around me. When I have hurt others, I've had to feel the shame and guilt that comes after my actions in recognition of the impact I've left behind. That shame and guilt, as I have stated, compound the depression and anxiety already present. They take me from bad to worse. Feeding negativity with negativity, it's unproductive. It's not fair. And, again, remember please—it's not your fault that you have depression. But it is also crucial that you remember it is not the fault of those around you either—so be careful with them. Mistreating others will only bring you feelings of deep guilt.

A Small Possibility

If you are in professional counseling and learn along the way that your depression *has* actually been caused, or is perhaps compounded, by those you spend the most time with, that would certainly be a reason to separate yourself from that source. Otherwise, don't blame your depression on others in your life and don't take it out on them. I know that I have before. Always with those closest to me. And I feel guilty for it every time. We have a large punching bag hanging in the garage. That and long walks. Both help. My family cannot be my punching bag, nor do I want or expect them to be. Everyone has their own version of a punching bag where they can place their burdens. Find yours, and make sure it's safe. You will always feel better after you get whatever is in you out. And you hurt no one in the process. Wonderful outcome. Sometimes when I hit that punching bag to a point of sheer exhaustion and I expel every negative thought inside of me with each strike, I feel closer to normalcy. Normalcy is good. Normalcy is better than shame. As far as shame goes, as a man who wants to present myself as strong, I have already admitted I have been ashamed of my depression all of my adult life. I'm close to moving beyond that, and perhaps writing this book will help, although I admit I am publishing it under a pen name other than my own. Guess I am not as strong as I wish I was.

I'm Sorry

To my wife—who holds me when I am not here, who
tries desperately to find me and bring me back out.
Whose touch I cannot feel when I am so far inside and
hiding for nothing—nothing but this dark, horrible
weight that creeps up my back and pulls me down before I see it coming.
Still, hold me—always hold me. I feel you, I know you
are there, I know you are real, I know you are love,
I know you don't deserve this. I'm sorry.

CHAPTER 13

Son

Nothing is more wicked than the dark beast that
strangles me right now from the inside out.
My darkness, my quiet isolation, my security, my
desperation. It lures me from despair to false comfort.
Just stay, keep me warm. Cover me, smother
me, suffocate me and paralyze me.
Keep my child at the door where I cannot love him,
cannot hold him, and will not hurt him.

Feeling Sadness

Depression and sadness are not the same thing. People who do not suffer this affliction do not necessarily understand that. Depression can lead to sustained feelings of sadness and despair, but feeling sadness over something does not mean a person has depression—thankfully. I've heard staggering numbers of people now taking medication for anxiety and depression these days, and two things puzzle me. Why so many? And if so many do take medication, why are there still so many suicides? Even for someone who has survived the temptation of suicide, it is still scary for me to think about the potential reality of that desperate act every time the subject comes up. I am still here on this earth as I write this, and that is why I ask. So many reasons to stay here. The tears I cried when I lay in my bed thinking about how awful it will be to no longer see my children each day, that sadness was real. That sadness became the reason to stay. There can be love in sadness, because there is value and substance. Feeling sadness means you are alive. Being alive, feeling alive is what we all long for. It can just be very hard to see through the fog of those confusing feelings when they mix with the dark sadness akin to intense low periods of depression. It makes the level of difficulty in attempting to set aside sadness from deep despair the same as trying to separate raindrops from the lake once they have fallen. They are one.

Again, depression and sadness are not the same thing. The opposite of sadness is happiness, while the opposite of depression's despair is hope. One is closer to the surface, while the other much deeper and complex. Sadness is a temporary emotion, while depression is an actual state of being. That could also be said of happiness versus hope. The deeper a state of mind can go, the more inspiring *or* dangerous it can be. If you can survive and overcome despair one time, you will inspire yourself to do it again and again. If you cannot, it becomes more dangerous when it repeats. Will I fail again, or will I rise above? That is the place in the mind from where strength begins. A place where losing turns failure into growth and overcoming, overcoming turns despair into hope, and hope turns weakness into strength.

If you need more understanding about this section, I suggest you do this: listen to the song "Bridge over Troubled Water" by the original performers Simon and Garfield, and then listen to another version of the same song by the band Disturbed. Focus on the composition, intensity, and tone. You'll feel it—sadness versus depression. It's pretty clear, and no, it's not an exaggeration.

More on the Topic of Music

Much like movies, music can provoke reflection and emotion. Similar to watching movies, music can connect the listener to the intention of the performer. For those of us that are introverts, this relatability factor is a necessary part of our need as humans to connect. As many types of music as there are, so too are the purposes behind each individual style and each song. Different music for different moods. Music can affirm our feelings, lift our spirits, or—be careful—it can keep us down in darkness when we are there.

Treatments to Combat the Growing Impact

I manage my depression and anxiety and do okay in my life. I do better when I exercise more, but many times the meds I take make me too tired to do things above and beyond my job. Caffeine helps, but that tires me out ultimately too along with dehydrating my brain (or so I am told). Well, no one's perfect. As far as other supports or treatments for severe depression, I have never taken lithium or electroshock therapy, two treatments someone in my family has tried when his depression became more than he could manage. I was afraid to look into trying those treatments, not because they seemed extreme but because they seem like last resorts. I don't ever want to be at the "last resort." That scares me because where would I go after the last resort? Death, of course. That's my primary worry.

I am still considering low-voltage shock therapy. I don't know what they call it these days, but I have read where others with anxiety and depression have used it and feel reconnected, clearer in thought, and even lighter afterward. Those are three specific outcomes I am looking for. I need to learn more about any new treatment first, but I am curious about it. Anything to make this life more manageable.

Hypocrite?

While I have mentioned my resentment over needing so many different medicinal supports to manage my depression and anxiety, my innermost desire for myself and those around me is still to get better. I might be willing to try new treatments, despite relentless complaining and resentment over needing them. If that means I'm talking out of both sides of my mouth, then I guess I am in this case. Sorry, that must be a part of my nature I haven't figured out yet. Perhaps a part of my ego I haven't overcome.

B.L. IYVER

Level

Lighter than before, level like anyone wishes they would be.
I remember the mood distinctly, but I cannot
capture how it felt to be down just days ago.
Depression is a horrible thief of normalcy.

CHAPTER 14

Wife

Nothing is harder than feeling nothing and appearing to feel everything
Holding you is holding everything
Holding you is holding life
Holding you is holding deep love
Holding you is knowing I feel
Feeling you is feeling me
Feeling me is knowing I am not nothing
You are everything—my life, my sense of knowing love, my ability to feel

Timing Matters

For me, the advice and input people give me usually only holds as much weight as where or who it comes from. Show me the research!— In reading this book, you could ask the same. Why then should you listen to me or anything I have written in this book? That's a legitimate question. You do not know me and likely never will. But by this point, you do know I struggle much like some of you. I hope that undeniable fact holds some merit for consideration with you. That the things I am sharing can lead you to some honest reflection inside yourself and, when you are ready, to action on your own behalf. Maybe my advice is good advice. Maybe parts of my list of strategies can be among your list and part of your plan for survival. That's the thing for me, the individual steps to coping with depression all had to be on my time line. They had to be proven to me, by me. They didn't necessarily come from others or their research. I am almost thirty years into this story of battling depression, so I would offer that my life *is* the research. I know enough about myself to know that the timing is right for reflection only when I decide it is right. You have to decide the same for yourself. That is something that is hard, if not impossible, for others to understand. Others close to you may not understand the timing piece. It will always seem to them, especially those who care about you, that the best timing for doing something about your situation is *right now*. This is the moment. Now is the time. I think that sense of urgency comes from others wanting to help and so "right now" feels like progress, feels like a step in the right direction, feels like they are doing something good for you in the time they have available to spend with you on any given day. Helping is important. We are not the only ones in this situation that feel helpless. It is hard for others close to us to fail at helping us when we are noticeably down. That can get frustrating for others. At the same time, if someone trying to help you gets frustrated and presses you by asking, "Why don't you do something to help yourself? Don't just sit there!" You may have to tell them, "I am fighting for my life right now. You just can't see it."—And then let it be. People cannot understand what they cannot understand.

My Wife

My wife has felt helpless many times. I can't imagine what it feels like to be her, to be a great wife and friend, to be everything I could ever want in my soul mate, and to feel that perhaps she is not enough. She must feel that way when I am at my lowest and weakest points. Perhaps if she was enough I would not experience depression? I hate that she probably asks herself that question. I am so blessed to have my wife. Why should I have depression with her in my life?—It's one of the confusing things that perhaps cannot be answered. I have worked very hard in communicating to my wife that my depression is not caused by her, but cannot be cured by her either. I believe it took a good ten years for her to understand that. That is very important. If I did not make that clear to her, time after time, she might carry the burden and that would be too much for any spouse to withstand. Yes, I am one of the lucky ones. I am married to someone who did not abandon me when my depression, time after time, surely made her feel abandoned by me.

One saving grace between my wife and I may have been her bout with postpartum depression after our third child, for which she needed medication and counseling to work through. I often wonder if that gave her just enough understanding about the challenge of depression to understand that sometimes you just have to step back and let the other person struggle. Step back but still love. Like Parker Palmer stated in his book, the person who helped him the most was not among the people who visited him often to have discussions, trying to motivate and help him shake the blues, or trying to get him out and about for a walk in the sunshine and around other people. Rather, it was the person who just came and sat with him and simply rubbed his feet that helped him the most. No conversation, no pep talks, no urging him to shake off those blues and get moving. Those silent foot rubs helped him as much as anything could at that time. The point is, it is *being there* that sometimes helps the most. If your partner can be there with you despite feeling like a useless failure for not being able to lift you up, that is a good partner and friend. Make sure you let them know how much you need and appreciate that. It matters. It helped me to survive. I am quite certain my wife despises my depression and the way it weakens me, but she has also grown to understand it better over time. Fortunately, she does not despise me. I know that has to be enough. I never give up, and she has never given up on me.

We All Need an Angel

Everyone has someone they owe their life to in one way or another. For some it is a parent; for others it is a grandparent or a best friend. For me it is my wife. I would not be here today if it was not for my wife. I thank God every day for her, in good days and bad—even when we argue and fight. After this many years, we find ourselves knowing how lucky we really are to be together. She is, and always has been, what I believe to be an angel that was sent to save me so that I could live out my life's purpose. She is an angel who saved me from myself. I am still here because of her. That is my situation; it may or may not be similar to yours. I would say, though, for those of you reading this who do not suffer from this affliction but are living with the person who does, I know you struggle just as much—only in a different manner. I'm sorry for your pain. I'm sure your loved one is sorry too, more than you may ever know. I spend time in prayer for my wife consistently because I know she must need it. Prayer can provide what I cannot. If you are the significant other of someone enduring a life struggle, we know it is hard for you not to be able to make it go away. We know and regret that we are making you endure a struggle of your own. We know you are not immune and nor can you keep your children safe from it—all things only my wife could understand in my situation. Perhaps someday she will write about how she survived all of this too—all the years, all the ups and downs, all the fears of wondering if I would hang on when she left me in that dark bedroom alone so many times. I cannot say I know how any of it is for her or my children for that matter, and I don't pretend to think I know. I have always hoped my children do not know what I deal with, but the older they get, the harder it is for me to conceal my struggle. I don't know how to share it with them or at what age it is appropriate to do so. I don't want to put any ideas into their heads about depression or anxiety, and I am not convinced that sharing my situation will be helpful to them. I would think having a professional help with that type of sharing and selecting the best timing and method would be smart. I'm not personally ready myself. Maybe that's a topic for a different book.

Do My Part

Having a dedicated partner in life is obviously very important. But my wife can only stay committed to helping if I do too. My wife knows I have never given up. I have not rejected medical treatment, counseling, or any other thing I knew could help. While I was at my lowest, yes, I was shortsighted and stubborn. But as I started to come up each time, without fail, I agreed to seek help. "You need to call the doctor" went from being something I resented hearing from my wife to something I accepted. I'm not sure I would say I have learned to appreciate those words, but of course, I do appreciate her care for me deep inside. It's just when that statement comes from my wife at the wrong time for me, as in during an argument, it doesn't help. Example: wearing my muddy shoes through the house once or twice while working outside on *our* house all day doesn't mean I need a doctor. Advice to loyal partners: in the midst of verbal conflict that has nothing to do with your husband's depression is not the time to tell him he needs to see a doctor. Relating this back to my experience, I would offer—throw other things at me if you want, just not that statement please! In calmer moments, when my wife may see me showing signs of an impending dip, is in fact the time for her to say it—and for me to listen. I have to own that. If she was not there to tell me, I may not even know I am slipping. If she had not been here with me all these years, I would be not still be here at this point. If you have someone in your life who cares enough and respects you enough to be honest with you when you're not doing well, hang on to that person and be a good listener. Commit to doing your part; you owe it to yourself and your family.

Disconnected

I'm starting to feel it—isolation, desolation, disconnected.
No anchor, no point of reference out, no path
paved to walk up and over into light.
Like quicksand, except without the comfort of the warm
sand encapsulating you like a winter blanket.
No, this is cold, dark nakedness—alone, not even air around me.
Please touch me, caress me, hold me so I can be certain I am still here.
Tomorrow I will awake, but to what?
It is a terrible thing to go to sleep in fear.

CHAPTER 15

Tired

Tired, who could ever be so incredibly tired?
Heavy, lazy, like a sloth.
This was never me, how could this be me?
How could I allow this to be me?
But you see, this is the me I pushed down inside
for too long. The strength it took to
keep you inside for so very long has now come to pay.
I am so very tired, almost too tired to even care. But I
know I need to rest and grow strong—strong enough
to stop pushing you back in, strong enough someday to
know you—to know me—to relent if even a little.

How Does This All Help?

You are fairly deep into this book now. Maybe something has resonated, but maybe it hasn't. I would offer the following perspective. There are books you can read that tell you how to fix, build, or accomplish something. Those books are put together more like manuals, and they provide a step-by-step process for the reader to follow, whether it's fixing your stove, building a deck outside your home, or carefully planning recipes for losing that extra weight you've been carrying around for years. The approach in those books is presented as exact and proven. This is not one of those books. Readers looking for solutions won't find one foolproof recipe here.

Yes, I've shared my own plan for survival with you, but that is *my* recipe. Be careful not to expect it to be yours. I hope that statement is not experienced as a disappointment, because I know right now you don't need another loss or another failure. That is not my intention in writing and sharing these memoirs or my plan for surviving depression and anxiety. Quite the contrary, I am sharing because I have personally experienced the incredible hope I feel in the face of relatability regarding my afflictions. Although the reality is a sad one and the flagrant reminders are discomforting given the bitter nature of the commonalities shared by those of us with these conditions, reading about them through the accounts of others does help to know you are not alone. And knowing *that* matters because one of the most difficult parts of having depression and anxiety is the compounding and potentially suffocating desperation of finding yourself alone. Being alone is dangerous, even in those low times when you may have intentionally sought isolation. We *must* grieve our pain, but we should not do it alone. The double-edged sword of isolation marks the difference between being alone and being lonely—and whether by choice or through necessity. I've always said, and told my own children, it's okay to be alone as long as you are not too lonely. Loneliness, for those with depression or anxiety, can be a terribly destructive force. Solace and solitude are not always kin.

Relatability through Vulnerability

My hope and prayer is that this book helps others by providing relatability through honest and transparent vulnerability as well as grieving our mutual pain and suffering. It hurts to hurt, plain and simple. I don't know what it is worth or actually why it has worth; but relatability has been, for me, a saving grace and sometimes so very important as a key ingredient to maintaining hope. Hope cannot be underestimated. In my lowest times of depression, I could not recognize feelings of hope but I knew it was there somewhere nearby. I grew to learn that during those low times, it was not only hope I could not feel. I could not, in fact, feel anything. Therefore, I was not, by definition, "hopeless" during those bouts. I was, instead, just completely numb—overwhelmed with nothingness—empty. Simply put, I was not there. It was during these times that I realized I needed something of substance I could reference that would provide context and clarity. Whether it was something I had written in my better days or something written by another, I need a reliable go-to when I cannot muster the ability to think straight on my own behalf. Hopelessness can take too many directions, try to at least steer yours. Hopelessness, I believe, necessitates acknowledging, feeling, and grieving your condition in the moment. That's something for me to remember next time I am down low. Perhaps I can look at my time in bed more as "good rest" than hopeless or hapless.

Poetry?

I went back today and read some journal entries I wrote during the many times I was captive to my bed for days at a time, and I was amazed at what I read. First of all, the writings are intensely real so I was not sure I wanted anyone to read them but me. I must say, though, they do a damn good job of expressing what it can be like to be there—sliding down, sitting at the bottom, or even rising back up from the lows. Some of the best poetry we all know often came from a time of suffering for the writer. Just like some of the greatest classical music compositions, the most beautiful paintings, or the grandest sculptures. My journal entries may be a poetry of sorts, I don't know. What I do know is that human suffering creates great works. History proves it. What I am pleased to say about my "poems" today is that I do not have so much sadness and shame about them as when I wrote them, that I no longer have to keep them hidden as I have for these many years. I am less ashamed of them than I used to be. If anyone else can read these emotional poetic writings, feel a sense of relatability and stay alive longer somehow because of it, then I will feel their purpose will have found its place.

A Star Is Born

You can debate whether the original or the remake is better. The original is almost always better. To my surprise, I actually thought Lady Gaga, or whatever her real name is, and Bradley Cooper did well in this film to convey all they hoped to. The topic of suicide in this film was quite real to me as was the path and the portrayal. Specifically, I watched that look in Bradley Cooper's eyes when he made the decision to cash it all in. To give up, to give in. To put down the hat for the last time. To take the final step that he (his character in the movie, actually) had already envisioned so many times. Despite love found, dreams realized, the world in the palm of his hand—he decided he had to go. Finally to be able to rest. To stop hurting and to stop holding others back. To stop sucking the life out of others in order to keep his own life going. To reach such a state of strength and resolve that an act of suicide becomes a stoic, manageable act, void of the panic, emotion, or the human instinct to survive that could prevent it in the final moment. Of course, I'm sure alcohol and drugs can get you there. Fortunately, I don't know what it is like to go through with it. I've always found a reason not to. There are so many good reasons to stay—so many. They are there if you just look. I encourage you to look for these reasons and to keep your focus on them.

Going Down Again

No!
No—not now, not again.
Whatever I did, I take it back. Whatever I should have done, I'm sorry.
Give me another chance. Tell me what I did to make this
happen this time. I'll never do it again. I'll add it
to the list.
Like all those other things, I'll never do it again.
How long before there is nothing left that I
can do without summoning you.

CHAPTER 16

Mid-October

*The leaves begin to turn. The temperature cools off to a
comfortable stage. And all the while, behind every
phase of the moon, the days grow shorter and the sun
grows scarce. Again I wonder—will depression bury
me again this winter like a heavy snow, or will I stay
above it with some sort of magical snowshoes. Such a
metaphor. But most don't know what it feels like not
to be able to stay above. Winter is coming and
nothing I do will stop that. Longing for the joy of Christmas
as when I was a child. Fearing for the depth of
depression I have known in more recent winters. This
trepidation is much more terrifying than Halloween,
I'll tell you that much.*

Winter

I could not write this book without acknowledging winter. Winter
is beautiful, fun, and wonderful; and winter brings Christmas!
Christmas is my favorite time of the year. I have always dreamed of
giving my family a good Christmas, and I think I have done so for
all these years. The fun of reliving childhood with snow forts, skiing,
sledding, snowball fights, and building snowmen! And Christmas
Day, such a celebration! Those wonderful parts of winter make it all
worth living through it with your own kids and, while you're at it,

working hard to stay in your marriage no matter how hard it gets so that you can build those Christmas memories together as a family. Those exceptional times also make it worth choosing to live, by the way. Think of all of the memories that would no longer be there if you were not there. Maybe it's time to take a break and watch *It's a Wonderful Life*. Sometimes, in the dead of winter, it is the memories that get you through the rough times until a day comes when more happy memories can be made. Christmas is the best of all things. But Christmas, to me, is not winter. And living through true winter, that is definitely no celebration.

Winter is what happens *after* Christmas. Winter is the series of bleak, barren months of cold and lonely existence that follow December. Between Thanksgiving and Christmas is a time of busyness and celebration. I'm too busy to get down, too busy to let up. Life through Christmas, and even until New Years, is usually pretty good. Then comes the letdown—the crash. January, February, March, and...sometimes even April. It can be a true punishment for those of us with depression. Specifically, winter depression can be incredibly difficult. It is putting life on hold when life is meant to be lived. How people living in the latitudes of places like northern Alaska ever survive their even lengthier winter season is beyond me. I understand why people live in the southern US, what joy and relief there must be in not enduring the bitter cold and darkness day after day. Here in the Midwest, I practically hibernate in the winter. Go to work, get home, eat, snuggle in, and go to bed. Wake up tomorrow and do it again. That's not much for living, but it is still better than dying. I do not know if there are more suicides during warmer months or during the cold of winter. If I had to guess, you could tell what I'd say.

I went to a tanning booth for five years during the winter months to try and help my winter blues. I also felt I looked healthier with a little color. Then I found out those tanning beds can supposedly give you cancer. So I am tanning to help me, in essence, stay alive; and that action could give me cancer that could kill me—really? Anyway, I stopped the winter tanning thing last year. But I may go back someday. I also have one of those special lamps you can sit and look at in winter to get the daylight you need in order to keep from sinking too low, but I am not sure if it does what it should or not. It certainly doesn't hurt, I guess. I work out and take Vitamin D3 in the winter too, so I am definitely trying—trying to give myself the support I need to stay mentally healthy and clearheaded during the long winter months. If you can muster the energy, exercise frequently in the winter. It can really help. And get your sun! Remember, the sun shines in the winter too. There is usually a window somewhere in the house where the sun warmly shines through during the winter. Sit there, close your eyes, and just bake in it. Ahhh...

Summer

Spring is so short that I can't even dedicate a section to it, not even a paragraph. I am not sure what happened to spring, but it seems winter just goes right into summer now. And summer, well, summer is the best of all times. Sunshine, relaxation, people, activities, outdoors, a better work schedule, recreation and play! Summer is a gift. Summer has held less trouble for me in my mind than any other season. Summer is forgiving, warm, and comfortable. Aside from a couple summers where my work gave me too much pressure, I have not struggled with intense lows during the summertime ever.

Being aware of how summer works for me, I once saw summer as a permanent solution. *Move to "summer" year-round*, I thought. Sunny Florida. The summer was good. The sun, the water, the dolphins! But when we did that, we eventually realized other things had been forfeited. Family, friends, Midwestern values—all back home. So as we started a family, back home to grandparents and the Midwest we went. Summer year-round will have to wait now until retirement. That's when people get the best of both worlds, you know, if they have worked hard enough to make it possible. I hope that's in my future.

Forgive me for a moment, but let me take this opportunity to divert this topic for just a brief minute and insert a related and important thought. As I write this section, I know today is a good day and I want to explain why. It is winter, and I am not questioning today and tomorrow. I am even looking ahead twenty years to retirement. Today is a day I not only want to live, but I feel I *am* living. The sun is shining, there's a light breeze, and my work for today is done. I wish I could make every day like this. But that is not my reality. My depression is with me still. It is just leaving me alone today. I could try to figure out why by looking at what I ate yesterday or today, how much I slept, what happened at work, and a hundred other variables—but I've spent enough of my adult life doing that already. That is time I cannot get back. In fact, I wish I would not have spent so much time and energy all these years trying to figure out my depression and anxiety or expecting them to go away. For me, at this point I am better off accepting they are with me and part of me. For you, I say you will have to determine this for yourself over time. Be honest with yourself and be forgiving of yourself—especially in the winter months. Summer will come—eventually.

Creeping Up

Summer—rest, family, sleep, sun
What is happening—what the f!% are you doing!?*
There's no pressure right now, no sleep deprivation,
no deadlines, no darkness—
what the f!% are you doing?*
I feel you creeping up.
Thanks a lot, these few months I have and
you want to take them from me?
—or are you just reminding me you could if you chose to.
I feel you creeping up, but I don't know why. Your
creeping up, though, implies you are in charge.
That bothers me the most.
I am glad it is summer, I have the will to fight you—and I will.
I think maybe I'll creep up on you—you useless f!%.*

CHAPTER 17

Not How I Feel Right Now

Too late. At least it's comfortable here in bed—
alone. I'm lucky, I got to hug all three of my
boys this morning and I know it's all very much worth it.

Mondays—The End of Relaxing or
the Start of Purpose Applied?

Winter has some issues, yes, but Mondays—they come all year! I am
not sure when it happened, but at some point Mondays became the
all-out enemy. It is amazing how much anxiety can build up into
Sunday night. Waking in the middle of the night to think through a
frenzy of concerns can be an awful punishment. And this can range
from perseverating on all the tasks that seem too overwhelming to
manage in the day ahead to a total attack with the locked stomach,
sweats, and all-out panic. Anxiety can be a dreadful, dreadful thing.
Worriers know it is hard, because anxiety is, simply put, illogical
worrying that has no direction, no solution, and no end. All you can
do sometimes is wait it out, or face it if you can muster the effort
and have the ability. What to do? Try to move through it. That's one
approach. And then the next time it comes on, you will be able to say
to yourself, "I got through this last time. I know I can do it again."
But depending on the level of anxiety, I know I've found myself completely incapacitated more than once—whatever the issues may have
been. I felt terribly desperate and deeply frantic inside my mind. I

just wanted to escape from my own thoughts. Over the years, this has happened more on Sunday nights going into the work week than on any other day, hands down. I started wondering if I should just start going to work on Sundays to work my way into the start of the week sooner! After all, maybe having Saturday off was enough for me. I should have taken notice when my coworkers gave me the comical magnet that read, "Work-a-holics anonymous, thank God it's Monday." What does that say about me? It says I put more value into work than play, and everyone knows it. So weekends weren't always weekends for me, especially after I gave up drinking. Staying busy took precedence over relaxation and reflection. While work has its place, it shouldn't be a substitute for healthy living. I recommend you take a different approach for yourself—if you still can. You won't regret taking weekends as actual weekends.

Diving into Work

A busy mind is a good thing as long as it isn't at 3:00 a.m. in the morning. That 3:00 a.m. awakening is the anxiety, front and center. I hate it. It is as terrible as it is uninvited. It is likely some of you know exactly what I'm talking about. If it's happening a lot to you, by the way, you either need a higher dose of medication or maybe a different job.

Someone very wise who must have gotten tired of listening to my woes about an impossible job situation finally said to me one day, "Just quit—there's always a different job." Well, it can't be that simple, especially if you have a family, house, and bills that aren't going to wait just because you want them to. It's not that simple. It can't be, right? Well, in truth, I think it *is* that simple. And it's true. There is always another job. But I've also learned you need to have your head together before making that type of change. If you have lead time, do every-thing you can to get level mentally and emotionally, plan out your finances for the transition, and then make the change. Remember, don't change everything in your life all at once. If you're changing your job, that's enough change at one time. When people try to change too much at once, I think that's often when people fail. They fail by expecting themselves to have more internal capacity for change than they actually possess. It is then that a tragic outcome such as suicide can result. No job, no income, no light ahead. That's a tremendously hard position in which to find one's self. Maintaining all other "normals" can be key. If you are going to make a job change, plan as much as you can. Reduce your bills and your monthly expenses. Make sure your insurance and medication are set to carry over so that they don't lapse. Changing occupations may mean taking a job at a lower pay level, a simpler role. But if it is for the sake of maintaining your sanity, it's definitely worth it. Choose humility over death. You can always build your way back up over time in responsibility and pay at your new job, which will happen naturally if you are your usual competent self in your new workplace. Remember, any job is better than no job! If the job you have is killing you, do some planning and then walk away. Don't let it kill you.

Winter—Busy Work, Happy Work?

A busy worker can also be a healthier worker in the winter. I dive into work, keep busy, and stay engaged in what I am doing. This keeps me from having idle time, idle thoughts and worries. If I am engaged in the present, I have no time to worry about the future and, for that matter, no time to regret or lament in issues of the past. There is nothing wrong with working a lot, especially in the winter if you are like me and suffer your worst bouts with depression in the winter months. As I said, winter can be grueling! Stay busy, make money, pay the bills. If that is all you can manage at any given time, your family is still getting what they need in life and *that* matters a *lot*. Even if you struggle with your emotional state all of the way into spring, as long as your family has what they need, you have done well. If you live alone, it can be the same for you. Survive through the winter. And by spring, you can look back and see the bills you have paid off and know that you made it through another winter— two great accomplishments. As far as work goes though, don't work yourself too hard. Stay engaged, stay busy, but try to have a work-life balance if you can. I am not going to write about that topic because

I am not one to talk. I have no work-life balance, or so I'm told. Honestly, given the challenges I struggle with in such unpredictable fashion, I sometimes think I am lucky to even have a job, and so I will cling to it with gratitude and work hard in it as long as it cares for my family in the ways needed. This, I know I can do even if there are other things I sometimes can't. Meaning, sometimes depression can take away parts of me, but it cannot take all of me. I can still be there for my family in a very important way, and so can you. My dad was a provider. He did the best for his family that he could—struggles and all.

Being Driven

Workaholics are driven. Being driven is something I have always been. In a counseling session, a therapist once asked me an interesting question. After listening to me talk for about twenty minutes, she stopped me and asked, "Do you know that you are always, constantly striving? Everything you say relates to something you are trying to accomplish. Every single thing you say! Isn't that exhausting?" I had to think about that for a minute. But then my answer was quite simply, "Yes." It *is* exhausting. The realization in that moment was profound for me. That notion of constantly striving had never occurred to me before. To me that was just *existing*. Isn't it interesting how we can be blind to things about ourselves that are completely obvious to other people? She was right. I am always striving, always trying to accomplish something, always pushing forward, always on the go and, sadly, exhausted and still never good enough. Good enough for what? Good enough by my own standards, that is.

Perfectionism—Far From Perfect

Perfectionism: that's a hard road to travel. I don't wish it upon you. But if it describes where you find yourself in life right now, take pause. If you are constantly on the go and feel the need to be accomplishing something at all times, it may be too much. If you feel lazy in any single hour when you are not accomplishing something, you're probably not in a healthy place. I feel lazy when I am not doing anything, and that means I struggle to relax—that's a bad thing. Relaxing is important, and it has its place, even for hard workers. No, *especially* for hard workers. People may compliment hard workers for their strong work ethic, but they may also recognize them as among those people who drive themselves into the ground. That's no good for anyone. Depression is exhausting enough; don't add to it if you absolutely don't have to. Work hard, but try to play and rest well too.

Thinking about relaxation versus laziness is an important exercise. Knowing the difference between the two is more important. I will write about the notion of *purpose* in a future chapter, and then I will explain where relaxing and being lazy both fit together in one life just fine.

Slipping

Cold January
Nice fire, happy home
November and December were better this year—don't
know exactly why but I'll take it—gladly. No, very
gladly.
February is almost here, why am I feeling this way
now? I rested, I ate, I exercised. But I'm slipping.
That desperate feeling. "Here I go again."
Am I the perpetual victim?
Time to exercise again, damn it. I own me, not you.

CHAPTER 18

To My Young Sons

*My sons, I wish for you happiness, sadness, experience,
and fulfillment. I wish your happiness to be real
and all of your choosing. I wish your sadness to be that
of knowing love. I wish for your experiences to give
you fulfillment—that nothing of my darkest shadow
is ever granted entrance into your hearts,
your minds or your loves.
Leave this part of me behind. Don't ever accept it as part of you.*

Advice about Time

If you struggle from anxiety or depression, or both, while my specific struggles and my plan to manage them may not be yours, I do have some advice that could apply to us all. It is about making time. Not time to work, not time to relax, not time to party. I could have helped myself more in my life by anticipating that I would need to block time aside for the bouts of deep depression I would experience and the recovery I would need time and time again. People with other known physical health conditions that flare up require rest and recovery. Furthermore, I've noticed that people who are part of their lives, both personal and professional, usually know about their physical health conditions and accept their bouts and even support alongside of them during recovery. Diabetes, kidney stones, Krone's diseases, etc.—others are aware, and that can help. For me, my adult life with depression and anxiety has been different because I tell no one. I have always been ashamed of it, seeing the weakness in it that flashes like a neon sign exposing my vulnerability and my inability to cope. When I am incapacitated by my condition, I am like a wounded animal hiding in the brush hoping that no one will see me, no one will know, no one will prey upon me. I hate it. But I don't just hate it for me. At this moment, I have to come back once again to how much I hate the impact of my afflictions on those around me. My family did not choose this; they inherited it without choice. While some husbands and parents are happy-go-lucky, work hard and play hard, I am not that and so my family does not get to live on that lighter side of life as I wish they could. I do not model a balanced life very well, and so they do not get to learn how to live one—not from me at least. I am what you might call a non-example. I am sorry for that. But I know, and you should too, that I would be hurting them even more if I was not still alive and here. So, again, that thought of, *They'd all smile more and laugh more if I wasn't here*—it's not true. That's a major bottom line you need to keep front and center as you work through your own personal situation. Remember there are people in your life that you love dearly, and there are hundreds of memories that include you that are yet to be made. Therefore, think about making and taking time for your bouts. Also, realize it will probably be important to work for someone who understands and accepts the limiting factors you live with and that they come and go. But they cannot understand unless you tell them. You'll need to tell them at some point if you have to take time off work and you want to keep your job, especially if that happens more than once. If it's the right job, you'll know. Just don't take advantage of the grace you are being given. If you are given time, use it wisely and limit the length and frequency you are out as much as possible. Then when you are well, help them remember why they need you at work. Doing so will earn you more grace when your next bout comes.

Relaxation—Family and Stress Part 2

So in my life I did laugh as a child. I remember loving time with my friends during my earliest elementary school years. There was not always a lot of laughter in my household, rather it was a busy, uptight, and sometimes frantic setting. I am not sure if that is why I have grown up struggling so much to be able to relax, but I would guess that is the case. I would offer this: tell your kids they can relax in your home and that they *should* relax sometimes. There's a difference between relaxation and laziness. I just haven't been able to figure out what that difference is personally in my own life, much to my own detriment. Hardworking parents, try not to impose a judgment of laziness on your family. Kids should have chores, and they should work for pay when they are old enough, but when their work is done, they should be encouraged to relax. You letting them, and even suggesting it, will give them a healthier perspective on life. In my house growing up, it was not such a healthy climate. When my dad walked in the house, you had better be doing something. And that something was not ever equated with relaxation. No wonder my siblings and I preferred to spend time at our friends' houses as much as possible. You know what they say, all work and no play makes...

When I became an adult I still laughed a lot—during time with friends, from internal happiness with my life, from movies, from alcohol, and whatever else came along that amused me. Sarcasm was sometimes a fuel for fun, but that came more so with the alcohol. I still have some dry wit today, but I have curbed the sarcasm. My sarcasm decreased along with drinking—and thankfully with the end of hangovers. But I still feel very lucky. I have several reasons to be happy and find laughter without alcohol. Do you have something you can do instead of drinking to relax and unwind? I'm talking about hobbies, fitness, or even love. And...you need *purpose*. That's right—purpose. A purpose that aligns with your beliefs and values. Purpose can fill many voids. Purpose is important. Without purpose you can struggle with identity. Purpose brings identity. Without purpose, you can lose hope. Hope matters. Without hope, you will lose yourself. With purpose, you will find yourself. Finding yourself means knowing yourself, and knowing yourself means you can better help yourself. Helping yourself sustains hope.

In my long experience with depression, I have finally learned that there are significant things I can use to replace parts of my depression that make my debilitating bouts more seldom and less severe. Purpose is one such replacement.

Purpose and Serving

"Immerse yourself in the service of others, and you will find your purpose in life." I'm not sure who first said that but, boy, were they right. When you feel well enough, carve out some time to help others. It may not come naturally, so you may have to make a special effort. With my situation, I know my depression had the tendency to make me more self-centered, I believe toward the effort of self-preservation. "I need to focus on myself so I can take care of myself." I know for years when I felt well, I would be selfish and fill my time with everything I enjoyed because I knew in the back of my mind that sooner or later my depression would come back and take it all away again. I was selfish with my time because of that. As an introvert, I did not naturally pursue group activities and events because it was easier sometimes not to deal with other people, especially people I did not know. Self-preservation was a good enough reason to justify my withdrawal from social circles. And all the while, I wish I would have known that involving myself with other people would only help me. Unfortunately, that was not my natural inclination. I viewed socializing, without drinking, as some sort of obligatory commitment I did not want to make; so after I stopped drinking, I started avoiding people. Because that avoidance can eventually lead to isolation, I must advise you not to do that. Isolation is not your friend. If my friends liked me when I partied, they would like me when I didn't. After all, hopefully partying did not fully define our friendships. And as for new acquaintances, they did not know me any other way so it really didn't matter. They knew me in only one way. It was all good. Other people are good. Remember that.

Again, when you feel up to it, do something to help someone else. Start with someone you know or someone you don't. It doesn't matter, and it does not have to be a big thing. Intentionally helping another person will open you up. When you help someone else, you reach beyond your own self-preserving mindset and outside of yourself. If you have been suffering from depression for a long time, you may understandably be quite deep inside yourself by now. You may even feel you are not capable or worthy of helping anyone else. What you will learn is that a selfless act can lift you up more than you may anticipate. Selfless, helpful acts also create sincere, authentic connections with others because, whether you felt it or not when helping another person, they certainly did. And being in a position of helping another reminds you that you are capable of helping people other than yourself. Service to others and understanding the significance of others' needs lessens perseveration over one's self. If you don't feel you can manage in helping another person, volunteer at an animal shelter and help care for animals, even if it's only an hour or two a week.

Vocation

To take it a step further, if you can find a line of work where you are helping others, that can be truly therapeutic to a person with anxiety and depression. It may not be foolproof, but for me, it helps. I admit I have still had times when I feel so low that I could not benefit anyone else, but I would like to believe that because I have chosen a line of work that serves others, my struggles have decreased in proportion to all of the good I am doing. If you have a different type of job to sustain yourself and your family that is not necessarily based in serving the direct needs of others, that's okay. Find ways and time to volunteer in service outside of work. Serving is helping. Like being busy at work, serving others takes your mind off your own issues. Take the focus away from yourself and put it on others. It can be quite liberating.

Fitness and Diet

Fitness and diet can be your two best friends. My diet is inconsistent. I am an adult man who, at times, eats like a teenager. Fast food and snacks. With how badly I want to cure my depression, you would think I would try to eat what has been shown to help with depression and stay away from things that don't. Well, sometimes my enjoyment in life comes from what I eat. Cravings, carbs, sugars. Our brains crave it. For those who would say, "Well, just change it then"—believe me, I wish it was that easy. It should be, but it's not. I know what you're thinking: *How bad does this person want to help himself?* Alas, I place more weight on top of my already heavy heart when I feel disappointment in myself. Be careful not to do that to yourself as a habit. So what to do about it? There has to be a different way to reach that positive end with my diet and exercise, and I'm still figuring out what that is. I have already stopped allowing myself to do some big things in life that used to bring me pleasure (aka drinking), so taking away foods that give me pleasure won't leave me with much! After all, we all need to be able to enjoy some guilty pleasures.

Sidenote: Interestingly, during this time of coronavirus, it has been six weeks since I graced any fast-food drive-through. That's a good thing, but we'll see how I do in a few months when restrictions are lifted. Regardless, what I have learned is, everything in moderation. I'm working on it. If you can do better than me in this area, do better. Exercise and looking fit both make a man feel better in general.

"Man Sick"?

In terms of making big changes in life to my benefit, there's really only a couple consistent factors over the years of my adult life that I can point to that have helped me dramatically in terms of resetting my life habits and neither are things I wanted. Hmm…what can I say about that? How can the two things that helped me most in my adult life be unwanted and uninvited?

The first thing that helped me was getting sick, and when I get sick, I am *really* sick. My wife may say I'm "man sick" sometimes, but I would tell you that when I get sick, it's for real—even to the point of hospitalization. It is then that I often reprioritize myself, vow to change my diet, see things more clearly, and long for getting healthy in more ways than just overcoming the illness upon me at that particular time. Any responsible person, myself included, can tell you that you shouldn't have to be dreadfully sick before you are willing to look seriously at evaluating your life habits. If it happens to you, though, take it as a gift. Pay attention to it.

The second factor that helps me consistently, one that I often have not viewed as something positive, is taking prescribed medications that work to level me out. Being level is truly a gift. I cannot speak for anyone else, but when I am *not* level, I usually still perceive that I am. That can be catastrophic, depending on what occurs. When I level out, I can look back and see that I was actually out of sorts, out of normalcy, and sometimes out of line. Medication that allows me to function fully in all the ways I want and need is a gift. Recognize medication as that. Despite my resentment for it, I know I'd be gone without it. Gone.

So stay healthy, eat well, exercise when you can, and take prescribed medication. You'll never regret it.

Regret

Regret is an enormous chain around the neck
A heavy burden that cannot be undone and so
it cannot be lifted as long as it remains
Regret is wasteful because it focuses on what
was instead of what could be
Live in regret and set the concrete around your feet—you
will never go anywhere and you will live in misery
Learn from mistakes and move forward, there is
everything to gain and nothing to regret
Regret is not valuable because it can be applied to nothing
Knowledge from experience is valuable because
it can be applied to everything
Don't live in regret, change what you can today and every day after
Let the past go—mistakes, loss, pain, regret
Let it all go

CHAPTER 19

Fury

Don't mistake fury for strength.
Strength is what manages fury; fury is what kills strength—
the strength in me, the strength between you
and me. So strong, and yet so weak in the midst of all of this.
Fury ravages like a hurricane. Fury stands tall
like a dictator, while strength eeks away
with a regretful disguise, embarrassed and ashamed
that fury has stolen all that is good.
Strength is lost in the anger of the self-
righteous, and all that is good is gone.
Fury and rage are bred from the same mother,
suffocated in the bosom of indignation.
Fury and rage are brothers in arms.
Fits of rage leave paths of destruction.
Not all destruction can be fixed or rebuilt.
Think hard before you let fury lead.

Self-Righteous

When my medication is working, I am a reasonable man—reasonable to live with, that is. Before reaching that point in my treatment, I was more unpredictable and I can remember getting ugly more than a few times. My ugly self-righteous face surfaces when I am getting low and, at times, when I am manically high. That state of mind can be dangerous and unstable for me and for those around me. It's the "one step forward, three steps back" state of being. But when it comes to doing harm, there are no do-overs in life and no taking it back. Feeling self-righteous can be a terrible thing. In some people it is ego, pride, selfishness, greed, disgust, or even entitlement. In me, it's simply ugly and misguided. Once the cutting words are spoken from my mouth, they cannot be taken back or erased. Whether I say them to my wife or my children, they are words recorded in history. I will say it again: take the meds. Take the meds and stay level. Level means life is okay for you and everyone around you. Level means you are more careful with your words. That is what I want, then everyone is okay, and no one is harmed because of me. I want to give my family a reason to want to be around me. I don't want to be the elephant in the room that everyone tiptoes around. Do you?

You will always feel better when you are not saying mean things to others, especially those you love. Swallow your pride and swallow the pill. Truth.

Isolation vs. Me Time—Be Careful and Be Aware

I want to come back now to the dangerous tendency of depressed people to seek isolation. We all need time for reflection and people with depression sometimes get too much of it. Reflecting and isolating are not the same. Although you may be by yourself in order to accomplish both, they are two very different things. Isolation is a natural tendency for those of us who struggle with depression. Simply put, we often get that feeling of "I just need to be alone." It can happen a lot, and it's not healthy.

Personally, I am not necessarily annoyed by others. I more so feel at times that I am not fit to be around others. Sometimes I cannot function. If I am isolated, I don't have to deal with anything or anyone. Sometimes that escape is just what a person needs. Even people without depression or anxiety need to isolate now and then. We call it needing some "me time." Most people see the value in it these days. Emotionally healthy people get some me time and then jump back in the game. Depressed people, on the other hand, isolate in sustained me time, looking to avoid issues or responsibilities of the day, hoping somehow they will disappear or magically be attended to if one isolates themselves long enough. The only problem is, everything a person is isolating from is still usually there when it is time to emerge. Emerging is necessary if you want to keep a job, a family, a relationship, and more. Be careful that your me time doesn't turn into avoidance time.

Moving Beyond the Morning

Throughout this book I share some poems I wrote during various states of depression. I wrote them in isolation. Once you read them, you will realize what I have realized in my life: that depression and isolation are unpredictable mates. Depression lures you into an escape from the triggers that cause your issues—or at least that's what it seems like in the moment. In other words, while depression is the problem, it can very well also present itself as the solution. Depression can be like a warm blanket, protecting you from the cold and giving you hospice from the cruel world outside the safety of your bedroom. Take my word for it, depression and anxiety have no intention to let you get up in the morning and get on your way. They'll keep you down for weeks if you allow it. Here's some advice: don't ever get comfortable in it or with it. Isolation is a slow path to suicide. Find a way *not* to isolate, at all costs, even if you feel you cannot cope with anybody or anything. Find a way to get out and to be around people. You can go to the library, gym, park, sporting event, or a hundred other places where people are, where life is happening, and you can be there without actually having to interact with anyone if that would be too much for you at a difficult time. At least you are around other people. Now don't get me wrong. There have been, and will continue to be, times when I cannot stomach any interaction with others. In fact, sometimes even when I want desperately to move into my day, no matter how hard I try, I cannot mobilize myself. I simply cannot manage it. I've become pretty adept at knowing when I need a day of separation and rest. Letting that feeling exist for a day is acceptable, but after one day it is no longer acceptable. Rest for a day. Sleep the entire time if you need, but when day two comes—get up and get out. Call someone if you need help getting going. If you don't want to talk, then message, text, or write an e-mail. That can make you feel just enough of a connection to get going on that day. Remember, I am speaking from twenty-five years of trying different approaches. I have discovered some very simple but good approaches. Please trust me enough to at least try once or twice. Send a simple text. The reply starts a conversation, and then you are outside of yourself and past your first obstacle. Some mornings it can be that simple to get going.

Without fail, when I have a rough morning but am able to move into my day and get to work, I look back at the end of the day and honestly wonder, *Why was it so hard getting going this morning?— Why all of that anxiety?"*—I am generally in a much better place at the end of most days. I try to remember that when the next difficult morning comes. And they will come, invited or not. It's, unfortunately, a guarantee.

Remember, the sun always returns in the morning. The next day always comes, with or without you, so it might as well be with you. The day is waiting, and fortunately, it's never as hard as your anxiety leads you to believe it's going to be. That's a really important thing to be able to tell yourself in those tougher mornings. It's very valuable for you and anyone else who is depending on you.

Leave

I feel you leaving.
I love when you leave.
When you leave I come back.
When you leave, cloudy days aren't another reason
to hate life, they are just cloudy days.
When you leave, a snowy night is beautiful,
not cold, dark and inconvenient.
I am grateful when you leave. What is it that I do to invite
you back? If I knew that, every cloudy day would
be easier, every snowfall would be beautiful.
Do I really need you to come so that I appreciate more when you leave?

CHAPTER 20

I can do all things through Christ who strengthens me.
—Philippians 4:13

So What Does God Have to Do with All of This?

We come to the part of the book where I need to say this:

If you do not believe in God, that is not a reason to stop reading. Please keep reading anyway. I am a Christian, but even I take time to learn about other religions. There is great value in understanding the faith perspective of others. Great value and wisdom.

For the greater part of my life I did not understand the Body of Christ. Although I contended that I believed in God, I did not know God. I was not a true believer. But for you, please consider this. It does not matter where you are in your faith journey right now. If you are an atheist, Buddhist, Muslim, Hindu, or any other religion, I still encourage you to keep reading. No one is trying to convert you, and importantly, this chapter brings together some very key concepts and practices from previous chapters of the book that, together, have led to my survival. Remember, this book is about surviving with depression and anxiety. In terms of converting people, this book does not aim to do what only God can do. There are pieces of my experience that can nevertheless be helpful. Anything that brings clarity to you can help you get back to making your list—your plan. So I hope, and I pray, that you will keep reading this chapter.

Two-fers

I was not raised in a religious household. We were what people call two-fers, meaning we went to church roughly two times a year—on Christmas and Easter. I was confirmed by a Methodist pastor in middle school after memorizing some Bible verses and going to confirmation classes for a few months, but I did not learn at that time about what it means to be a believer in Jesus Christ. That was not likely the pastor's fault. I was not focused on what we were discussing during many of the class sessions. And we did not talk about it at home. I am just a lucky person because I met and eventually married someone who was raised as a Christian and a true believer in Jesus Christ. While I admit I kept her faith at arm's length for nearly fifteen years while we dated, married, and started a family, I did eventually get saved. That was God's will for me. It did not happen from classes, or church attendance, or one single recognizable event. It happened over time, bit by bit, as I realized I literally could not survive without God. I got to a point in my life where I gave up. I gave in. At least that's how I saw it. My depression had defeated me, and it had done so soundly. I failed. I was broken and weak. And so I turned to God. I wanted to live, and I prayed for help. I wanted to have a life with my wife and children, and I wanted it to last. I asked God for help, and He answered.

God Answers Prayers

In recent years, I gave up control of my life one thread at a time and I have replaced it with faith and trust—not in myself, but in God. I leaned on others for wisdom and understanding as I learned about faith and trust. I asked others to pray for me and to teach me. I looked at serving in life a new way: not to "do good" and no longer striving to "be the best" at everything I did, but to act only as a faithful Christian should.

I accepted Jesus Christ as my Lord and Savior, and He saved me. I committed my time and my work to serving others, in the name of Christ. Remember what I said earlier about serving others.

When you focus your energy on helping others, you think less about yourself and you feel only goodness about helping others. It's a win-win. There is no room for negativity or constant worry. They just don't fit.

I have my wife to thank for leading me in this direction and for not giving up on me. As I wrote earlier, I believe she was an angel sent to save me from myself. She must be incredibly strong to accomplish what she has. She also relied on God. And our marriage is still surviving today, which is also a small miracle.

Nothing Easy

I always thought if I reached a point in my life where I let go of my vices and turned to God, my life would at least get easier. It might be less exciting, I predicted, but it would at least be easier. All things in goodness, right? For the record, being saved did not mean "life got easy." My life got better, yes, but to my surprise, it actually got harder too. As a believer, my life is *harder* now than it was before. But how can that be? My life was hard enough already. Please let me explain. As a believer, my faith is still challenged daily. My battle with depression and anxiety has shifted to a spiritual battle. I believe there is good and evil in this world, and as my faith grows stronger, so too do I recognize all of the growing darkness in the world around me—including my own. I am a sinner. Consider that I had spent the better part of fifty years as a type A perfectionist. Being a believer means accepting myself as I am. And, like all humans, I am a sinner and I am most certainly flawed. Accepting this is nothing easy.

I'm Not Perfect

As a person with strong perfectionist tendencies, accepting myself as a sinner meant accepting that I am wrong, flawed, and imperfect. That hurt. But I have grown to understand that what has hurt me even more was trying to be perfect for all of those many years. If you are one of those unfortunate souls that strives for perfection, please do yourself a favor and let it go. By doing so, you'll be doing a great favor to yourself and those around you too. Luckily, I got to a point in life where I just didn't want perfection anymore. Honestly, I couldn't take it any longer. Always holding too high of expectations, always setting myself up for failure and disappointment, always walking right into the trap of unreasonable expectations and away from my humanness. My perfectionism, whether it came from within me or grew from early expectations placed upon me, was a key ingredient in causing my anxiety and depression. I truly believe that. Therefore, I try very hard not to impose that tendency upon myself anymore. And I am also careful not to impose it on my own children. If you have children, please think about it. Perfectionism is painful and merciless, and you would never want to be the cause of pain for your own children. Remember, the only perfect being to ever walk this earth was Jesus Christ. He was perfect, so we don't need to be.

Long-Suffering

As I shared, my daily life as a believer is a struggle. But it is not the same debilitating struggle of depression and anxiety. Yes, they are still with me, both of those unfortunate conditions; but my faith does help me to better recognize and manage them daily. It's been a long road, but I have lived and learned. Through faith, I have learned about the long-suffering, praying, and the act of asking for patience in affliction. Having the ability to recognize suffering as a part of a natural human path, rather than an insurmountable static obstacle, has given meaning and release to several of my recurring burdens. So many incredible examples in the Bible, my own struggles pale in comparison to what the believers of old endured for their faith in Christ. And my small worries, they are nothing compared to what matters in a world with Christ.

Purpose in Suffering

Nonetheless, I bring up this topic because it is precisely the understanding of the notion of long-suffering that can help those of us challenged by depression to better navigate through it. The long-suffering has a purpose. Remember, purpose is good. Purpose provides direction. Purpose takes us outside of ourselves. Purpose makes a person whole. People who feel whole feel mentally and emotionally better. Get it?

The Struggle

In our culture, suffering is seen as something unfortunate and undesirable and struggle is often seen in the same light. Why is it that struggle is expected for marathon runners and Olympic athletes, but for the rest of us struggle is something we view as "bad"? Conversely, the Bible tells us that struggle is to be expected in life and that it is necessary and good. Knowing this helps in understanding the need and place for suffering in our lives. As a believer, I will suffer because I have to. Since Adam took the bite from the apple, we are all destined to suffer and struggle. But the Bible also tells us there can be joy and fulfillment in the struggle and even in the long-suffering. Joy can be more recognized in the midst of the suffering, like a ray of sunlight shining through a broken storm cloud. We are meant to suffer in life to some extent. That's right. As someone worthy of struggle, I can rejoice in my struggle because God is with me and He has already won the battle for me. This means I can relax a little. It's going to be okay. Life is going to be okay. God provides, so I can stop the worrying. I can let my anxiety rest.

Stop the perseverating and intense need for control. Stop striving at everything. Turn your work into service, and strive to be a faithful servant. God will provide; He always does. In knowing this, in truly believing it, anxiety is decreased. That is a gift beyond measure.

Faith or Medication?

There are schools of thought that say afflictions such as depression and anxiety can be cured through prayer and prayer alone. After all, God can do anything. That is true, but my own understanding is that God expects us to help ourselves as well. Does taking medication mean I am weak in my faith? I've thought about that often. I am fortunate to have a pastor who says, "You cannot just pray away your depression and anxiety. Pray, yes, but go to counseling and take the medication if you need it."—What a blessing to hear this from someone I feared would tell me that prayer by itself should be enough. If someday I no longer need medication, I will certainly pray in gratitude. But today is not that day.

> *The Lord saved me from death; he stopped*
> *my tears and kept me from defeat.*
> *And so I walk in the presence of the Lord in the world of the living.*
> *I kept on believing, even when I said, "I am*
> *completely crushed," even when*
> *I was afraid and said, "No one can be trusted."*
> *What can I offer the Lord for all his goodness to me?*
> *—Psalm 116:8–12*

CHAPTER 21

Evil

*Sometimes I feel that my sense of the greatest love of my
own family is only truly known in comparison to
the deepest desolation that mirrors in opposition to my best feelings.
My darkness is evil. I know that it is because it shields
my outgoing love. I cannot feel love when my
darkness comes.
My darkness is real. It is evil. It is not perverse or wicked,
but it is certainly evil. I know this because it is not
borne of goodness.
It is evil, impotent sometimes, but evil nevertheless.*

Is Satan the Maker of Anxiety and Depression?

I thought of ending the book with the cheerful realization that becoming a believer has helped me tremendously with managing my anxiety and depression. While that is true, as a realist, I cannot negate the darker side of where my depression lives. Exposing it feels appropriate and necessary.

God didn't fix my depression or my anxiety. He helped me to see them more clearly and accept both in a manner that lessens their impact and their hold upon me. They no longer rule my life. They do not limit my life in ways that are so destructive as in years before. But they are both still here in me, and they can surface at any given time, on any given day. Is that Satan at work? I do wonder, but I have no clue. I really do not want to give him that much credit. Satan, to me, is the deceitful part of depression that wants me to give in. Satan is the warmth of isolation that fools me into feeling I am in a good place by myself. Satan is every temptation that leads me away from my purpose, and he is in every critical part of my nature that makes me despise the weakness I see in myself and others. Satan is fear, and as Zach Williams says, "*Fear is a liar.*"

Is it Satan that wants me to kill myself? I would venture to say yes, but it is not his fault or his privilege. Satan does not possess that kind of power. It is not Satan that kills anyone; he is simply the one who places the option closer within our reach. He seeks to comfort the afflicted in their weakest moments by offering poor choices that appear desirable, to guide the lost at their most venerable point in the wrong direction. He deceives. He yearns to keep souls from reaching God. Beware because he comforts suffering humans even to the extent of presenting himself as a false angel of Christ, or even bolder. I have read where Satan has even presented himself to ailing souls as Christ himself!

Ego and Pride

Satan also loves working through our egos. Satan stalks the prideful and the wounded and pushes them into further darkness with instruments of fear or temptation. All of his paths lead away from God and straight to hell. He will give you all that you desire. He will fulfill your wildest dreams, but remember this: nothing he offers or promises will ever be granted without a terrible cost that you will eventually and inevitably have to bear. Read the small print, as they say, because Satan is the master of deception.

Fear

Supposedly, over 75 percent of the decisions we make as humans are from a base of fear. Isn't that awful? Blame it on our survival instinct, our tendency for self-preservation, or perhaps on our lack of trust and faith. I blame myself, but I do not take full responsibility.

As a believer, I also acknowledge that Satan is around us and, as the Bible states, he is waiting to pounce like a hungry lion. The Bible is very clear on that. The evil one, as he is often called, loves when we are fearful, unsure, and lacking in faith. Those are some of the things that give Satan his strength. After all, it is our own free will that gives in to Satan's ways instead of choosing God's, oh we of little faith. But you do have a choice. I have God in my soul because I invited Him in. I am a part of the Body of Christ. I have no need for this fear and, thus, no need for Satan or any of the temporary luxuries he offers. When I place my faith in Christ over the fears and temptations invoked by Satan and all ungodly things, I have found the ability and strength to overcome the anxiety that has come over me so often. I excuse it. I let it move on, just as simply as I move on to the next order of business in my day. And the more times I dismiss my inclination toward anxiety, through faith in Christ, the less cumulative anxiety I have over time. Since I have been made to understand that my anxiety is what leads me into depression, as a believer, I now have a better fighting chance with both.

My Biggest Obstacle

Satan is not my biggest obstacle. I, myself, have always been the biggest obstacle in solving my own situation with depression and anxiety. When control did not work, I just wallowed in misery and waited it out. I tried to figure out what changes I could make, what triggers I could better recognize, and what steps I could take to make my bouts with depression less frequent and less severe. Don't get me wrong, there was value in that process as is evidenced by my list that eventually developed into a plan through that long process. However, I missed the main aspect of my situation for so many years. Listen carefully. Depression is not rationale, nor is anxiety. If either one is the result of a chemical imbalance of some sort, regardless of how that imbalance occurred over time, thinking your way out of it will not work. About six years ago I finally accepted that, and it was a Bible verse that kept finding its way in front of me that finally got me to see. I saw it on bumper stickers, church bulletins, and even on a billboard! Obviously, someone was trying to tell me something. Proverbs 3:5 says, "Trust in the Lord with all your heart, and lean not on your own understanding." That's right. Guess what, when you stop trying to rationalize everything, it will release an enormous burden from you and you can stop thinking yourself into exhaustion. Once you accept that, just let go and let God. Proverbs 3:6 says, "In all ways acknowledge Him and He will direct your path." Now see the two verses together and say them together (only if you'd like, of course):

> *Trust in the Lord with all your heart, and lean not*
> *on your own understanding; in all ways acknowledge*
> *Him and He will direct your path.*
> *—Proverbs 3:5–6*

Could it really be that easy? I would tell you, yes, it can be. Dare I bring one of my favorite bands, the Eagles, into this right now? Absolutely, here are some great lyrics—"So often times it happens that we live our lives in chains, and we never even know we have the key." Once you've adopted Proverbs 3:5–6 (and maybe the Eagles), I am not contending that life is easy, but it sure makes a lot more sense than it used to. Your burden can be much lighter; it's truly beautiful. To know that peace of mind is within your grasp is priceless.

Ending Worry through Prayer

Anxiety is a brutal punisher. I think we've covered that thoroughly in this book. The time wasted in worry is Satan's pleasure, plain and simple. An effective and reliable tool to end anxiety is prayer. Someone I respect persuaded me to take everything I worry about and stop perseverating on it or, conversely, trying to push it out of my mind. He said I should just adjust my middle-of-the-night self-dialogue from worry to a self-dialogue of prayer. So I tried it, what did I have to lose? I took each worry as it came into my head, no matter how fast or furious, and I prayed about it if even briefly.

I prayed to God, and miraculously, I found a wonderful result. As I wrote earlier in this book, the worst thing about waking at 3:00 a.m. with anxiety is that by 6:00 a.m., when it's time to get ready for work, I am already mentally exhausted. I am beaten down, and I feel I cannot cope with what lies ahead in my day. As I understood it from my wise friend, I needed to pray about being able to lay my worries at the foot of the cross. I had to pray to let go of them. "God, I give you my worries and my anxiety. Please take them from me." Some nights I would pray one thing after another, for two to three hours. I was skeptical but hopeful. Then one night, about a month after I started replacing perseveration with prayer, something amazing happened. After starting into prayer at 3:10 a.m., the next thing I knew I awoke to my alarm at 6:00 a.m. I had fallen back asleep. Not only had my prayers been answered with restful sleep, but after a few more weeks of prayer I started to notice that the concerns I laid at the foot of the cross through my evening prayers starting holding less significance during my days. I prayed more, and as I did, I became better at it. I started to enjoy it quite a bit, and I experienced results. The answers to my prayers were not always what I expected, but my prayers were definitely being answered. Good things started happening, and they did not feel coincidental. I was becoming a stronger believer.

People of faith will tell you, when you go from feeling you *have* to pray as an obligation to becoming someone who craves and looks forward to prayer, you are truly a blessed person. When you start to experience the strength of prayer, it is more powerful than any medication or anything else humans can accomplish. (No, I still couldn't stop taking my meds after becoming a believer and an avid prayer, but I *will* share that my doses are in fact all decreased and I'm still doing well. That's something. Let's call it a healthy compromise.)

Scripture

I mentioned previously that there is a movie or a song for every mood, for any type of situation. As a believer, I want to tell you this is even more true of scripture. That is a journey I would encourage any person to follow, but not one I will go into deeply here.

Religion Is a Crutch

I am smart enough to know that some of you are reading this and perhaps you don't buy a word of it. While I'm sorry to hear that, I understand. Yes, I used to be there too. I saw religion as a crutch. I did. For many years, religion just didn't connect with me. I observed that when people's lives got hard, they seemed to turn to religion. Not to God, mind you, but to religion. And it seemed to happen only when things went wrong. My thoughts at that time were as follows: *Religion is for the weak. If people believed in God they would turn to Him when they were basking in happiness—not just when things in their lives got bad.* I saw great hypocrisy in religion, especially in organized religion, and that was an obstacle for me for many years. I confused religion with knowing Christ.

As a believer in Christ and someone who prays daily to God, what I say today is something quite different than I did back then: "Forgive me, Lord, a thousand times over. Forgive my pride, my ignorance, my arrogance. I'm sorry. Thank you for my life. You give me more than I deserve."

Strength in Numbers

I am never alone. God is always with me. Even when I am isolated to the confines of my bedroom, beneath my blankets, incapacitated by the way I feel—I am not alone. And yes, that still happens to me once in a while but not nearly as often as it used to. Praying is powerful, and it does help. Spending one day in bed is way better than three or four days. I can live with that now and then. The next day always comes, and it is better. I pray, and my prayers are answered. I can move on, and I do.

I have asked God to strengthen me so that I may serve in the manner that He has gifted me. I hear a voice on those mornings when I don't think I can cope with the coming day, and it helps me to get up. No, I don't hear an actual voice that speaks to me in words. But I do sense a voice about me, around me. And then it is my own voice that I hear saying, "Get up!" But it is certainly God's supportive voice that guides my own. I leave my bedroom and my house, and I travel to my destination, unscathed and poised to lead by the time I arrive at my destination—free from the anxiety that was upon me only hours before. If anxiety is something you live with, on more days than not, you have to be able to have a greater voice than your anxiety.

Strength in Believers

Another support that helps me get up and go each day is knowing that—regardless of where I am headed that day—when I reach my colleagues, my family, or my church community, I know I will be among believers and their faith can carry me during the times when I am weak, just as my faith will help to carry them when they are weak. Together we are stronger. We are not in it for ourselves. We are, rather, in this thing called life together. There is strength in numbers. My faith and path as a believer has led me away from isolation and the dangers inherent in it. If you struggle, Satan wants you to struggle alone—with him. Say no.

There is wisdom in my experience and true growth from my struggle. Let me add one more element of strength that is worth consideration. I believe that, in the midst of people of faith, it is harder for darkness to manifest itself in my mind—whether it originates from inside or outside of me. The faith of many is an amazing shield of protection. There is no room for darkness in a brightened room.

Not Easy, But Better

My life is better than it was, but it is not easy. I still need to follow my list—my plan. Adding God to the top of the list has made the difference for me. That is not something I am imposing upon you, but as a believer, I will profess that God offers it to you. All you have to do is ask if, or when, you are ready.

As a believer, I do not cast my entire list of coping strategies out the window and place my expectations upon God. I believe He guided me in creating my survival plan. With free will, I choose to take medication, stop using alcohol, exercise, try to eat better, sleep as much as I need, see a counselor, let go of perfectionism, accept the struggle, love God, and—most importantly—I choose to never, ever give up.

Top of the List

For me, God is number one. He is the light and the life. And so now I can finally share my *completed* list with you—my proven plan for survival.

My list of strategies to live with and survive with depression and anxiety:

1) Pray to God. Praise our Lord and savior, Jesus Christ.
2) Take the medication—depression is a disease, not a habit or weakness you can break or overcome through sheer willpower.
3) Whether you are more afflicted by depression or anxiety, or both, set aside your pride, lay down your ego, and ask for help or you won't make it.
4) Stop drinking alcohol—period. And while you're at it, stop any recreational drugs you are using too. They are all depressants. Alcohol and depression don't work.
5) Go to work daily. Keep your job, your income, and your insurance.
6) When you are not working, remember the things you enjoyed doing as a child and start doing them again, no matter what they are. Your mind and heart will remember.
7) If your work does not involve service to others, find a way to serve others outside of work.
8) Accept and pay for counseling to understand two things: (a) it's not your fault and (b) depression is a condition you have to acknowledge in order to manage, not a weakness to be ashamed of.
9) Don't wear your depression like a banner, but don't hide it from those people who are important to you either.

Concealing it will crush you—and them. Flaunting it will drive others away.

10) Find healthy physical outlets. Pent up feelings can be dangerous to yourself and others.

11) Don't ever be fooled by the deceptive comfort of isolation.

12) If you are in a long-term relationship, let the other person know what you deal with. And never, ever hold the other person responsible for making your depression go away.

13) Don't ever give up, no matter how much sense it makes to you or how dreadfully exhausted you get. Know and accept that your depression and anxiety will come and go—possibly forever. Plan for it.

Believers Bonus:

14) Remember your blessings and count them often. You will recognize all the wonderful things you have instead of dwelling on those you don't.

15) When you've had a really bad day or a bad week, pray for a better one ahead. It will come.

I count on this list as a plan from month to month, week to week, and even day to day. I rely on this list when I am healthy and when I am in a state of disarray. Even in my lowest points, the list is something I know to be accurate. The proven experience of each item is foolproof for me. I know I can trust what is written here even if my struggling mind tries to tell me otherwise. It is therefore a plan of action. My list, within each separate item, has the ability to ignite healthy thinking and positive actions. It leaves no doubt about what does and does not work for me in surviving my depression and anxiety. I am able to stay alive.

Your Plan Is *Still* the Key

It would be great if my plan works for any of you, but as I said it is not intended as such. Work on your list, and don't stop until you finish it. The most important thing to remember after your list is completed is to trust it and refer to it at *all* times. If you swing down into a bout with depression, which may include loads of irrational thought, stick to the trusted words that you have written in your own pen. This will not only keep things from getting worse in your depressed state of being, but it can help bring you up and level you out sooner as well.

Make a plan and stick to it. In doing so, my bouts with depression and anxiety have become less frequent and less severe. I am living proof. I want this to happen for you.

Conclusion

As you've gathered by now, Will Ferrell didn't actually save my life, I guess, but he sure helped. Thank you, Will. As you've done for me, I am sure you have made many people happy, time and time again. Taking people away from their worries, away from their hurt and pain, if even for a short while, is your gift; and I am so glad God placed you in the role where your talent can shine and brighten the lives of all of the rest of us. Thank you for making me smile and laugh. Giving joy to so many others is true service.

In Christ Alone

I end with Christ. I could not find my way forward in this life without God and those who have led me to Him. I am immensely grateful. Perhaps your plan may lead you to God eventually, who knows. I would just offer this—depression is an uphill battle. If you think you can do this on your own, I'm not going to say you can't. I'm just going to say, you don't have to.

Live on, brothers.

Let Go and Let God

I am broken, imperfect and sinful.
I am tired, worn down and exasperated.
I am not in control and no longer seek to be. I am
not in charge and realize I never was.
I am not as important as I once thought.
Decrease me so that You may increase.
I am a believer, a person lost who has been found.
My burdens have been lifted. My sins I leave at the foot of the cross.
I am relieved; relieved of having to carry my burdens.
I am cured; cured from believing my life should
be without struggle or suffering.
I am saved; through His grace alone, I am saved.

For God hath not given us the spirit of fear; but
of power and love, and of sound mind.
—2 Timothy 1:7

EPILOGUE

About My Poems

Throughout the book you have seen my poems, or anecdotes, if you will. They begin and end most chapters. Written during my struggle, they may inspire you or bewilder you. Some are dark, painful, and confusing while others are joyous, unearthing, and more. When offering them for your view, I am a bit worried about how real these writings will be to some of you. My poems may be made of the same struggles that are inside of you. Some are written from such desperation, pain, and anger that the thoughts included in them may be dangerous. But they are real, and those anecdotes may just be written in a way that recognizes and acknowledges some of the similar pain and struggles you live with—enough so that they connect with your inner suffering so you know you are not hopelessly alone. Again, I believe relatability can be a saving grace. No one understands exactly how you feel, but knowing that others feel and anguish in ways similar to you may be enough to sustain you while seeking a better way to cope and make it through—or better yet, overcome. If my story is enough to persuade you to seek help, then I feel my suffering had a purpose and, for that, I would feel incredible gratitude.

The Grueling Context—to Those Who Do Not Endure Our Struggle

Although grueling, the redundant narrative and context of this book is quite intentional. In its totality, it is meant to offer relatability for those afflicted by depression and/or anxiety and a very clear and realistic lens for those who are not. It's as grueling as it appears in this book. The bottom line is, there is no brief or convenient narrative to depression and anxiety. There is great value and great empathy, however, in understanding the plight of others who truly suffer. People who suffer from depression and anxiety cannot survive without help from those of you who do not. We need you. Thank you for having the strength to be there with us and for us.

Life over Suicide

Our days are already numbered, brothers, God has already set forth the day we enter this earth and the day we leave. Within that time, our purpose is defined and what we choose to do with it through free will determines the rest. I urge you to let God be the one to number your days. Don't cut short the joys and triumphs He has planned for you in the days ahead. These are things of which you are not yet aware.

ABOUT THE AUTHOR

Author B. L. Iyver is a student of life, grown by God to become who he is today through years of victories, losses, triumphs, struggles, and a healthy balance of joy and suffering. Living the experiences of both small-town and big-city life during his lifetime, he has very privately battled depression and anxiety for over twenty-five years. Until being saved in the last decade, B. L. did not understand the purpose behind his experiences. Today he is coming closer. Through the gift of continued life he has received from God, B. L. feels compelled to reach out and share his story in an effort to try and help other men discover concrete ways to live out their lives and walk away from suicide, a horrific crossroad he has faced multiple times during his adult life. As a husband, father, and professional, B. L. understands how blessed he is in this life, hence struggling and anguishing to understand why he suffers as he does. Ashamed as a man of his condition, he strives at all costs to conceal his struggle for the sake of his family and his professional life. His shame and pride have collectively weighed him down to a point of utter exhaustion, defeat, and brokenness. A brokenness that allowed for rebirth. Through this book, B. L. Iyver hopes to expose and release his own burden of affliction as well as help other men by providing an intensely real and highly relatable account that helps them to know they are not alone. He has found that choosing life over suicide can be accomplished through properly managed strategies and habits, medication, and, most importantly, living through Jesus Christ.

Printed in the USA
CPSIA information can be obtained
at www.ICGtesting.com
LVHW091254110524
779935LV00002B/487